Acknowledgements

"The Magic Forest has been a proper adventure. Ten years in the making, editing and doing my very best to create the simplest system possible."

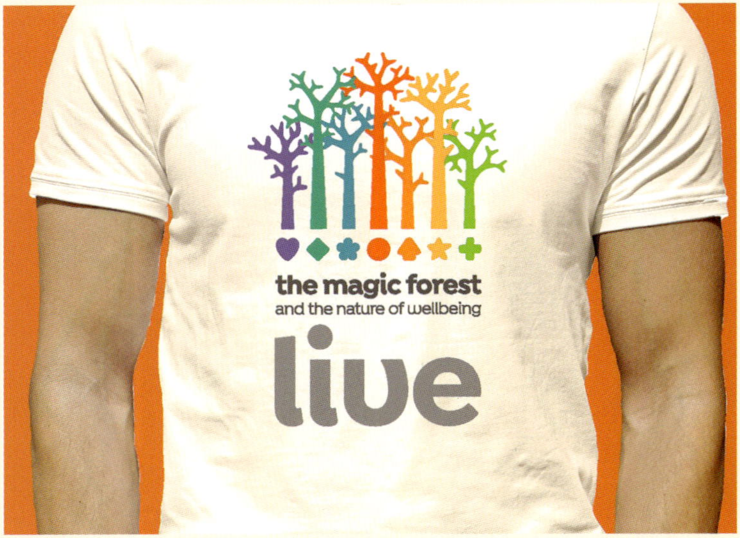

Acknowledgements and thanks to:

My parents who taught me to find my own voice and who sadly will never be able to read this now.

Max, Jodi and the Payne family.

All the friends and customers who patiently listened to my ramblings, helped and fedback.

Grayson & Philipa Perry for inspiration.

Paul and Bob for keeping me company.

The Magic Forest and the nature of wellbeing.

First edition: July 2023

ISBN: 978-1-7394657-0-4

Printed in China.

Published by: Park Designs
O S Homfray T/A Hammer Design
2a Hathersage Business Park, Heather Lane,
Hathersage, Derbyshire, S32 1DP. U.K.

Ideas & concept, author, layout & design, editor, art direction, illustration and typesetting: Si Homfray

www.parkdesigns.co.uk
www.hammerdesign.co.uk

Contents

hello + welcome

"Seven trees and forty nine words but not all necessarily in the right order..."

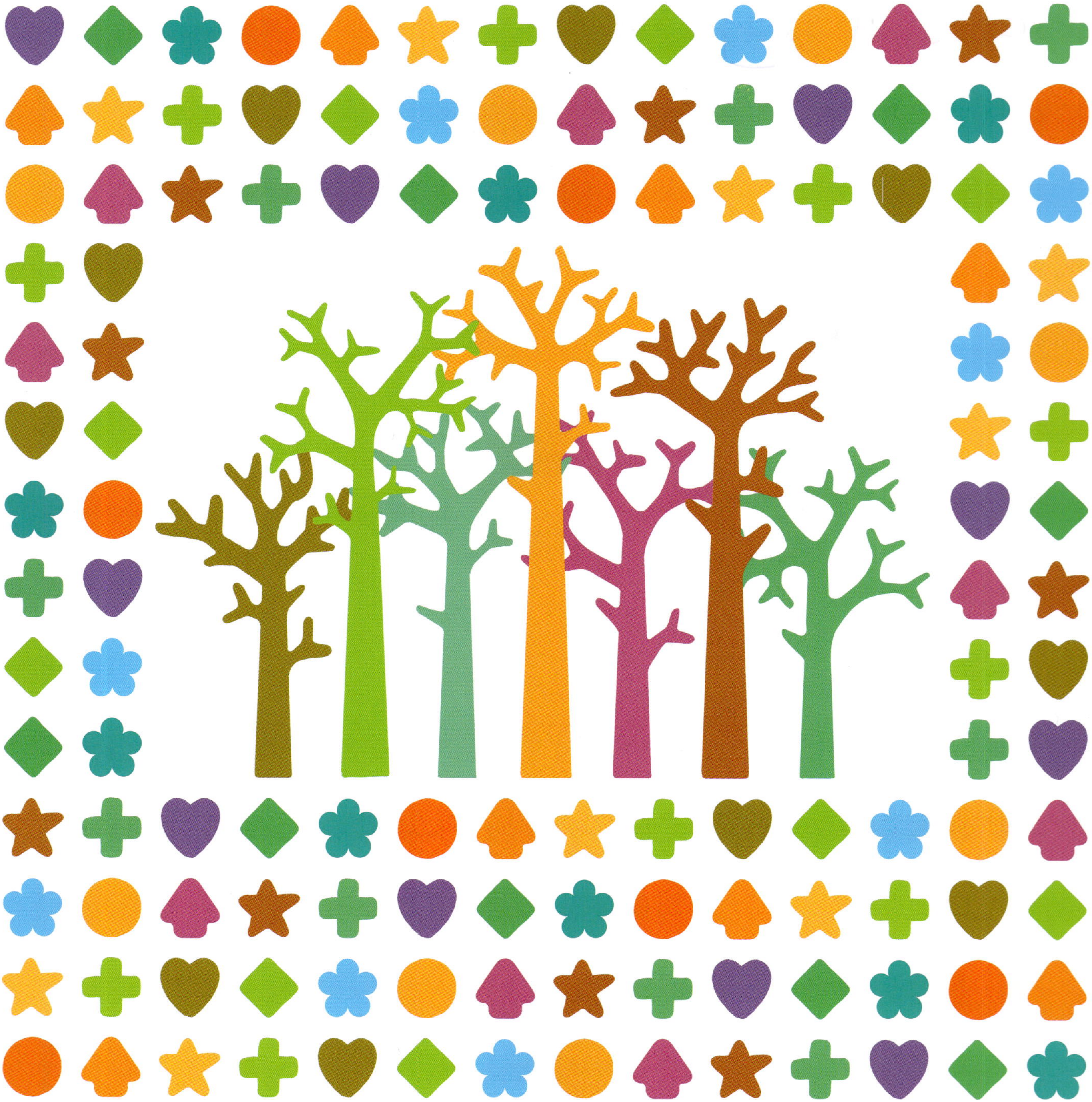

Preface

This book has been conceived, written, designed and put together over many years from the very best place.

The process has been cathartic and I am so relieved it is all over for the time being. The important thing to say is that it has been written from a position of warmth, not financial necessity, a personal need to find the simplest structure to pass on to my son, look after myself, make sense and make the most of... my life.

Frustrated by the plethora of material out there, and the complete absence of anything comprehensive that was presented simply, I persisted against the cries from friends and people who had a vested interest in my wellbeing.

So here we are, the first edition, perhaps of many, with the purpose of getting the system book out there as soon as possible to provide a framework for others' questioning as well as producing the ingredients for some new design and art projects for my future.

I really hope you like the system and find something of use. I certainly did. So all that remains now is to wish you all the most heartfelt best wishes in your personal growth and exploration, and for me to get back to some outdoor adventures and some serious arting. Yey!

Si Homfray 28-01-2023

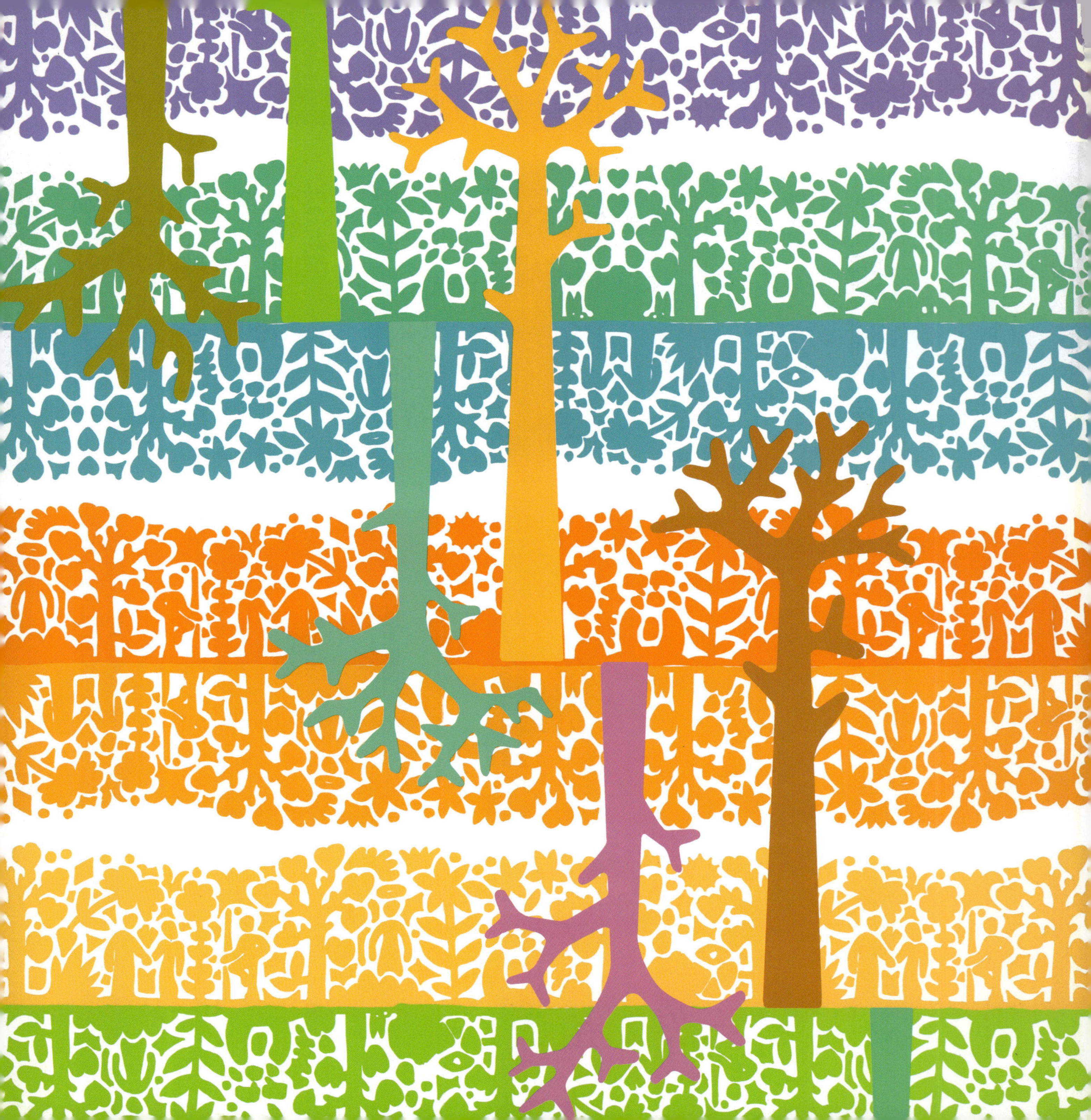

Introduction

This book is a simple visual system, designed to cover all the aspects of improving your wellbeing as a whole. One key area at a time.

There are seven chapters for the seven core trees that represent the most important areas of our physical and mental wellbeing.

These trees make up the Magic Forest and it is left to you, the reader to work your way through the forest in any way you choose, asking key questions and learning about yourself as you go. By using this framework with repeated questioning, eventually, you should build yourself a more solid foundation for a better balanced and healthier life.

The magic forest and the nature of wellbeing is a simple visual system for exploring your own wellbeing.

The structure is built around seven trees each with a set of seven words to work through.

The words and their accompanying questions, insights, quotations and challenges cover everything you might need to do in order to achieve a rock solid foundation for wellbeing and a **balanced healthy life.**

This is a big claim, but the simple system is both elegant and comprehensive, designed to allow the user to find their own way in their own time, through their own understanding and answers.

The keywords have been selected to encourage questioning, thinking and further investigation through the forest maze of both mental and physical health.

The system has been designed in as straightforward and as clear a way as possible, to allow shortcut insights into personal growth, and a useful structure for persons who find the plethora of contradictory health and wellbeing advice 'out there' confusing.

The concept, content, graphic design and illustration has all been designed for the modern world by si homfray.

'Collectively these words are amongst the most important words in all our lives'.

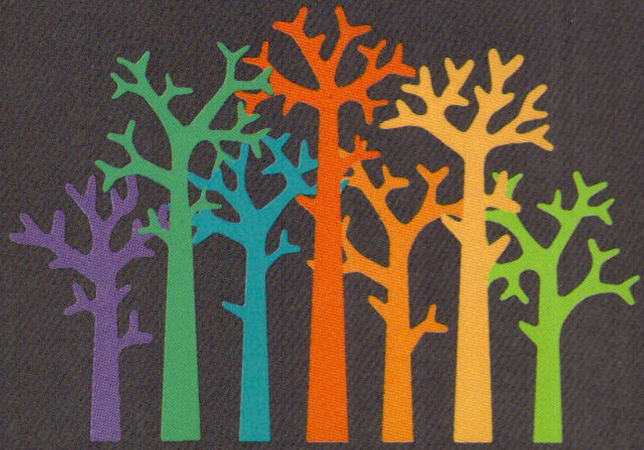

the magic forest
and the nature of wellbeing

the most succinct wellbeing book in the world today?

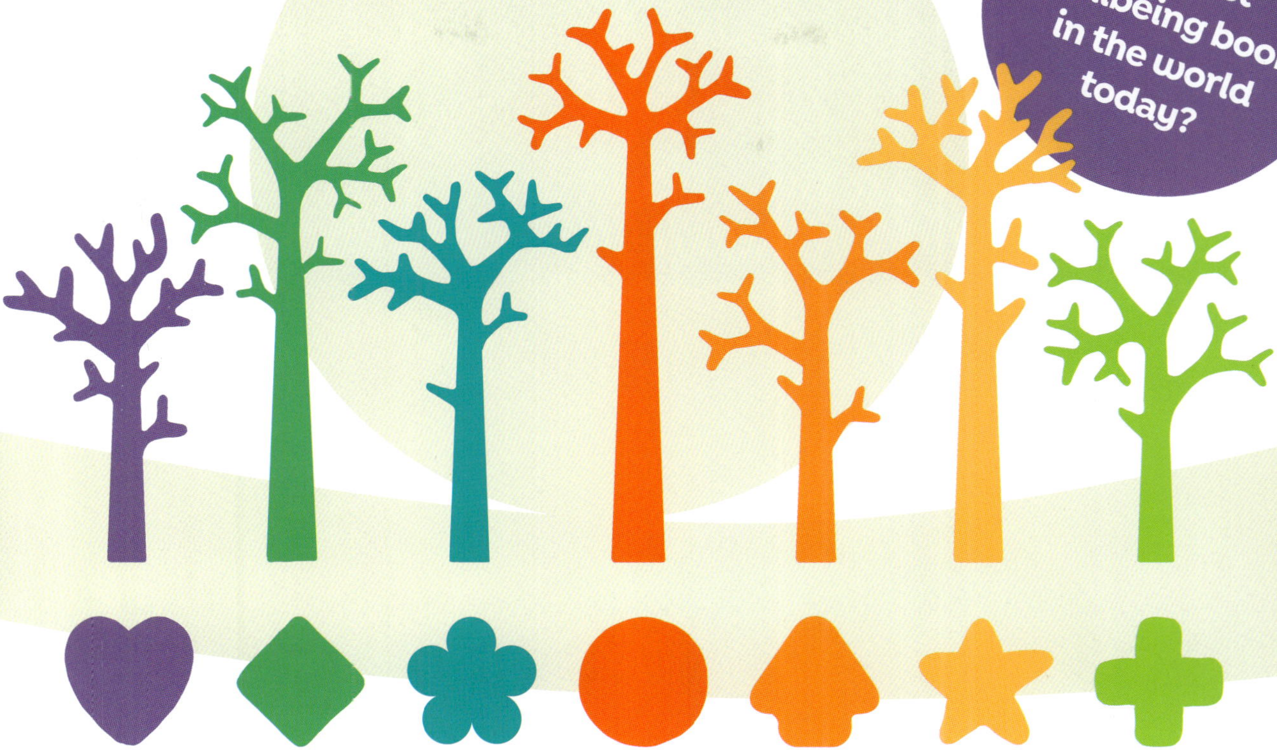

the magic forest

and the nature of wellbeing

7 trees, 49 words and a very abridged text.

How to use this book

The Magic Forest book is a framework, a set of keywords, to ask questions about yourself, this way you can find your own answers.

Ask questions and find your own answers

You can use this book in one of many ways: Skim read, dip in and pick a question to ask yourself or read one tree at a time.

Key

Interest or info.
Interesting relevant insights and information about the word and its relevant application such as a definition.

Questions to ask
The questions and challenges that succinctly ask and answer why should one should use this word as part of your wellbeing exercises. without prejudice or bias.

Benefits
The benefits and relevance of understanding and accepting the word into your wellbeing exercises.

Quotation
A strong summarised and ideally memorable quotation about the wellbeing word.

I really feel that these simple words, if used as a starting point to ask your own questions about your own life, can quickly answer so many important fundamental aspects for you.

The keywords provide a simple focus and a framework for looking at and understanding what you need to do for a more healthy balanced life.

'Revisit and repeat as many times as you like'.

In time by going around the words again and again, your questions will change and you will find and develop your own personal tools that assist the way you look at and deal with everything that goes into your wellbeing.

Given all our lives are different, you can take away what you feel is important to you. This will build the framework of who you are, your foundation of solid wellbeing with all it's different points, for your life as you grow.

“Building a rock solid foundation of wellbeing, one word and one question at a time”

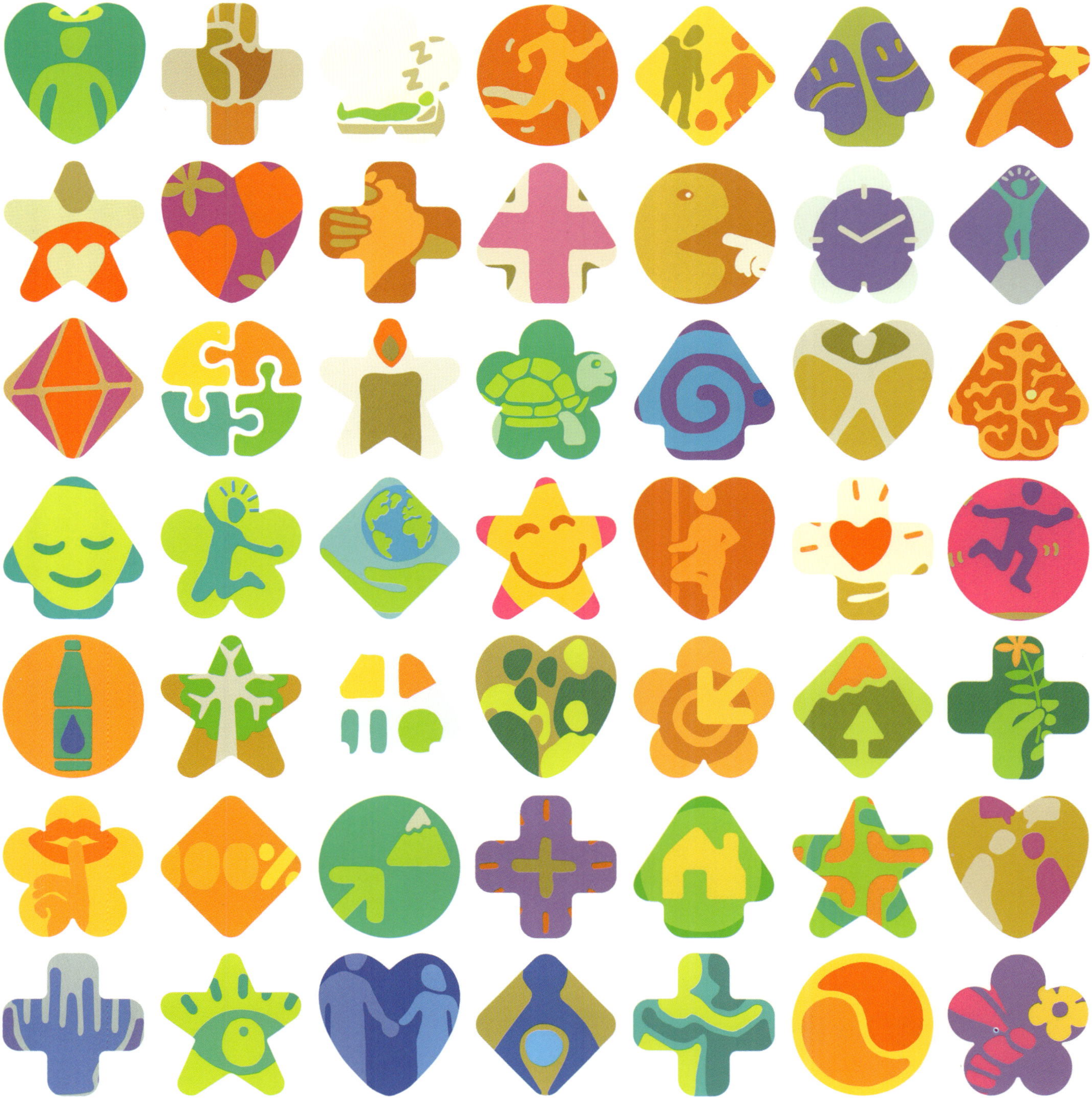

The 7 key trees

belonging

The Tree of Belonging - Your people
These words help build your wellbeing through a sense of **belonging**, love, communication and improving all the relationships in your world.

---

purpose

The Tree of Purpose - Your world
These words help you improve your sense of **purpose**, through an improved understanding of your needs and finding your place in the world.

---

time

The Tree of Time - Your time
These words help you develop a better wellbeing through an understanding of your time, living in the **now** and your rest and recreational rewards.

---

body

The Tree of Body - Your body
These words help you build a greater understanding of your nutriton, hydration, exercise, needs and motivation for a better **balance** for your body.

---

mindset

The Tree of Mindset - Your core mind
These words build your wellbeing through your **attitude** and approach to your life using a safe place in your mind to develop your understanding of how your mind works and can be controlled.

---

mindsight

The Tree of Mindsight - Your inner you
These words help you build your wellbeing by developing a better understanding of the way you and other people see your world, building an improved love for yourself through your **perception.**

---

self esteem

The Tree of Self Esteem - Your mind work
These words help you build your personal **confidence** and self esteem through a better understanding and improved interaction with other people.

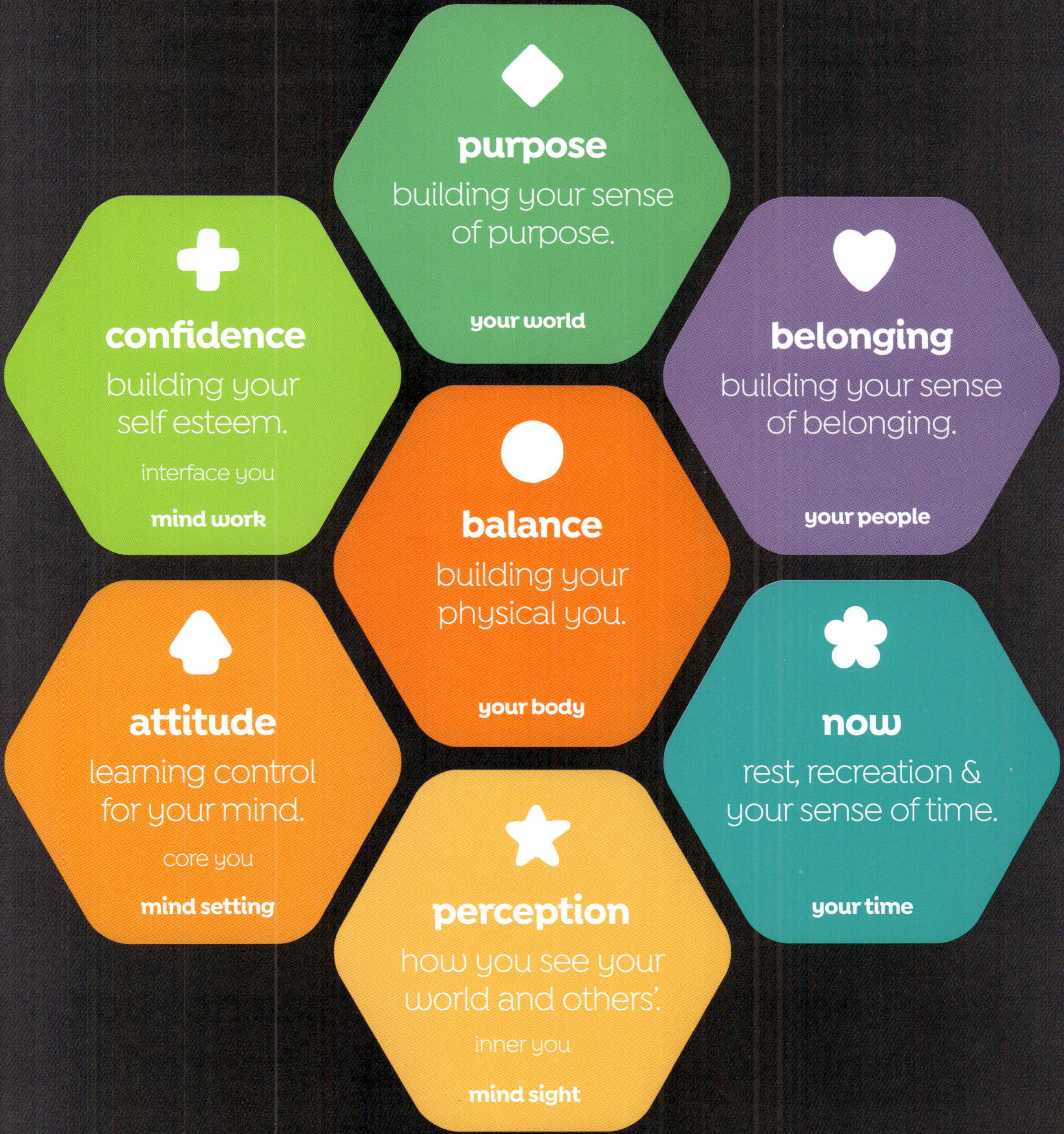
purpose
building your sense of purpose.
your world
confidence
building your self esteem.
interface you
mind work
belonging
building your sense of belonging.
your people
balance
building your physical you.
your body
attitude
learning control for your mind.
core you
mind setting
now
rest, recreation & your sense of time.
your time
perception
how you see your world and others'.
inner you
mind sight

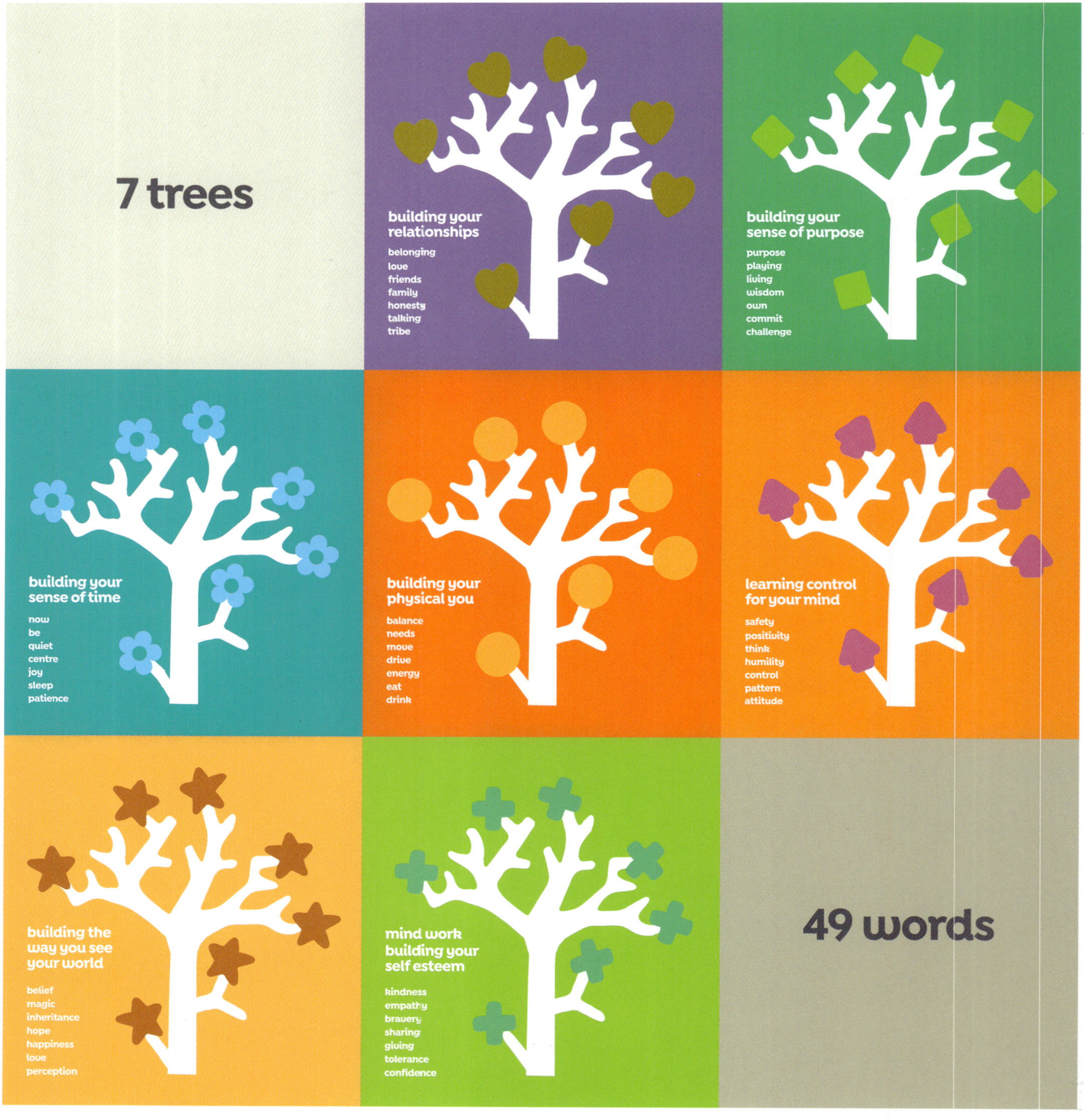
7 trees
building your relationships
belonging
love
friends
family
honesty
talking
tribe
building your sense of purpose
purpose
playing
living
wisdom
own
commit
challenge
building your sense of time
now
be
quiet
centre
joy
sleep
patience
building your physical you
balance
needs
move
drive
energy
eat
drink
learning control for your mind
safety
positivity
think
humility
control
pattern
attitude
building the way you see your world
belief
magic
inheritance
hope
happiness
love
perception
mind work building your self esteem
kindness
empathy
bravery
sharing
giving
tolerance
confidence
49 words

“Every great adventure starts with a first step”

The Tree of Belonging

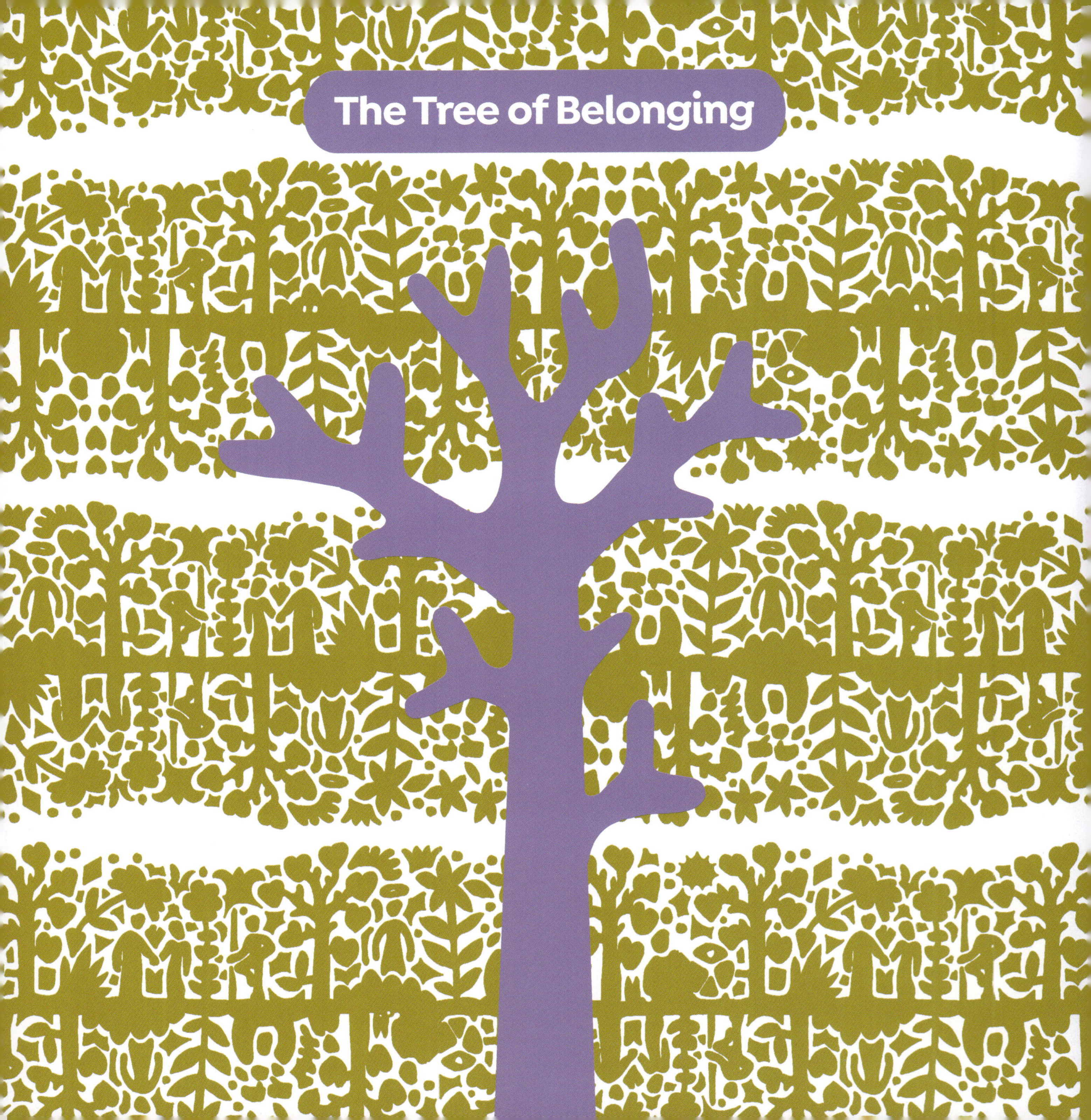

1

love

honesty

talking

belonging

building your sense of belonging

friends

family

your people

tribe

1 Your People

The Tree of Belonging is the first tree in the Magic Forest of wellbeing, and it is all about your people and building your relationships.

The words in this tree help you understand the work you will need to do to help build your overall wellbeing. Working with, talking to, understanding and looking at your relationships with all the people around you in your world will help you build your sense of belonging and ultimately improve your own feeling of wellbeing.

The following questions, quotes and insights are a summary of essential elements to help you build your relationships, finding your place in the world one action or one deed at a time.

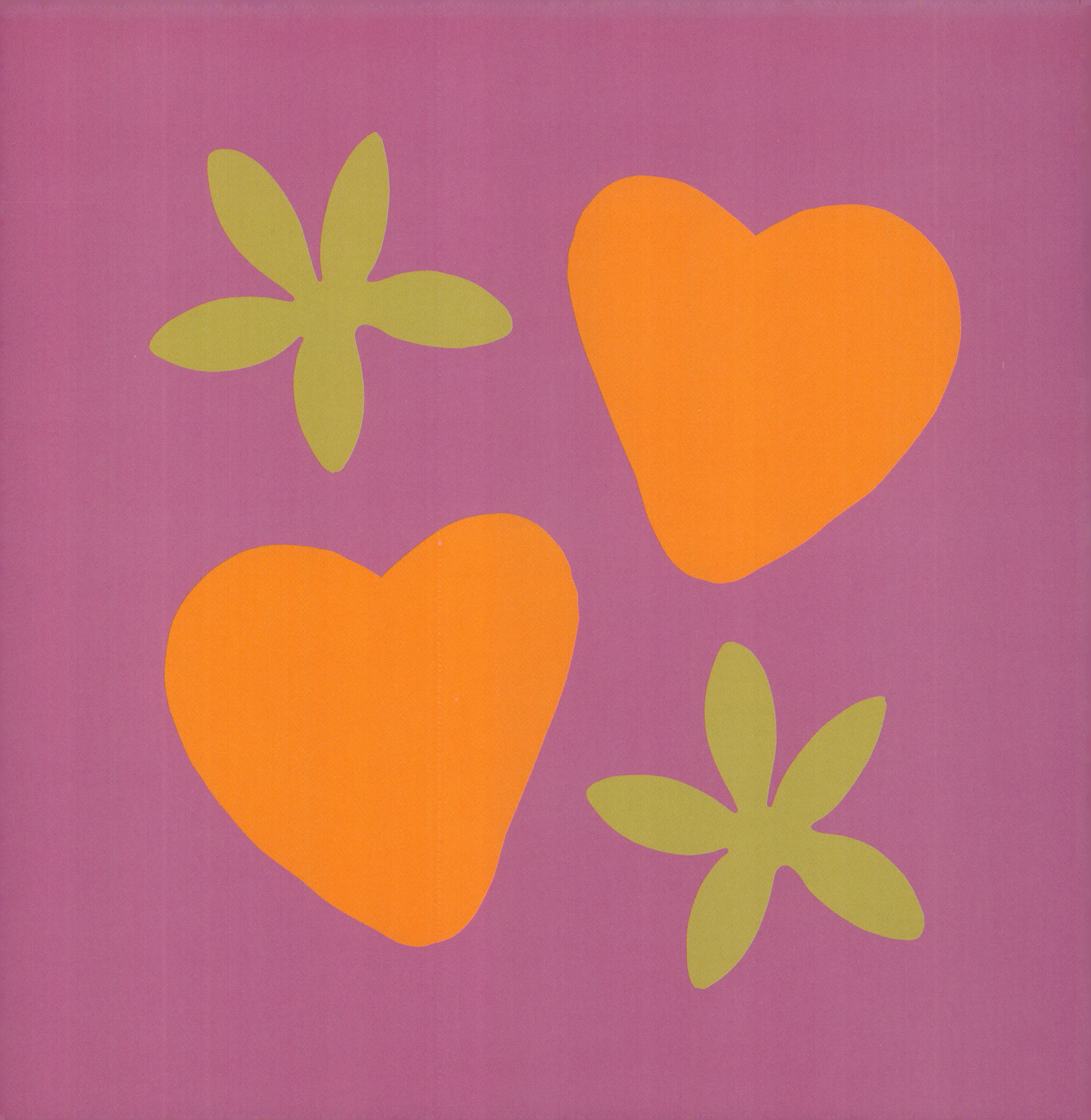

Love 01

Where love is present, relationships flower and bloom. Loving and being loved opens many doors on the path to solid wellbeing.

The worlds of cinema and music have written the greatest words on love, memorable phrases built into our language such as 'all you need is love' all of which go on to humble this author.

A good question to ask of yourself is 'How can I be more loving?' in the sense of kind, thoughtful and supportive to those around me. A greater and more challenging question might be to ask 'What is stopping me from sharing all this love I have to give?'

Loving someone or being loved, put scientifically, releases a great many chemicals and will release many physiological benefits for both the giver and the receiver. Finding **a loving approach to your life** and all the people in it is the big ask, building great relationships the result. This is at the very core of great personal wellbeing.

"Where there is love there is life." Mahatma Gandhi

"Love is the only force capable of transforming an enemy into a friend." Martin Luther King, Jr.

"Being deeply loved by someone gives you strength, while loving someone deeply gives you courage." Lao Tzu

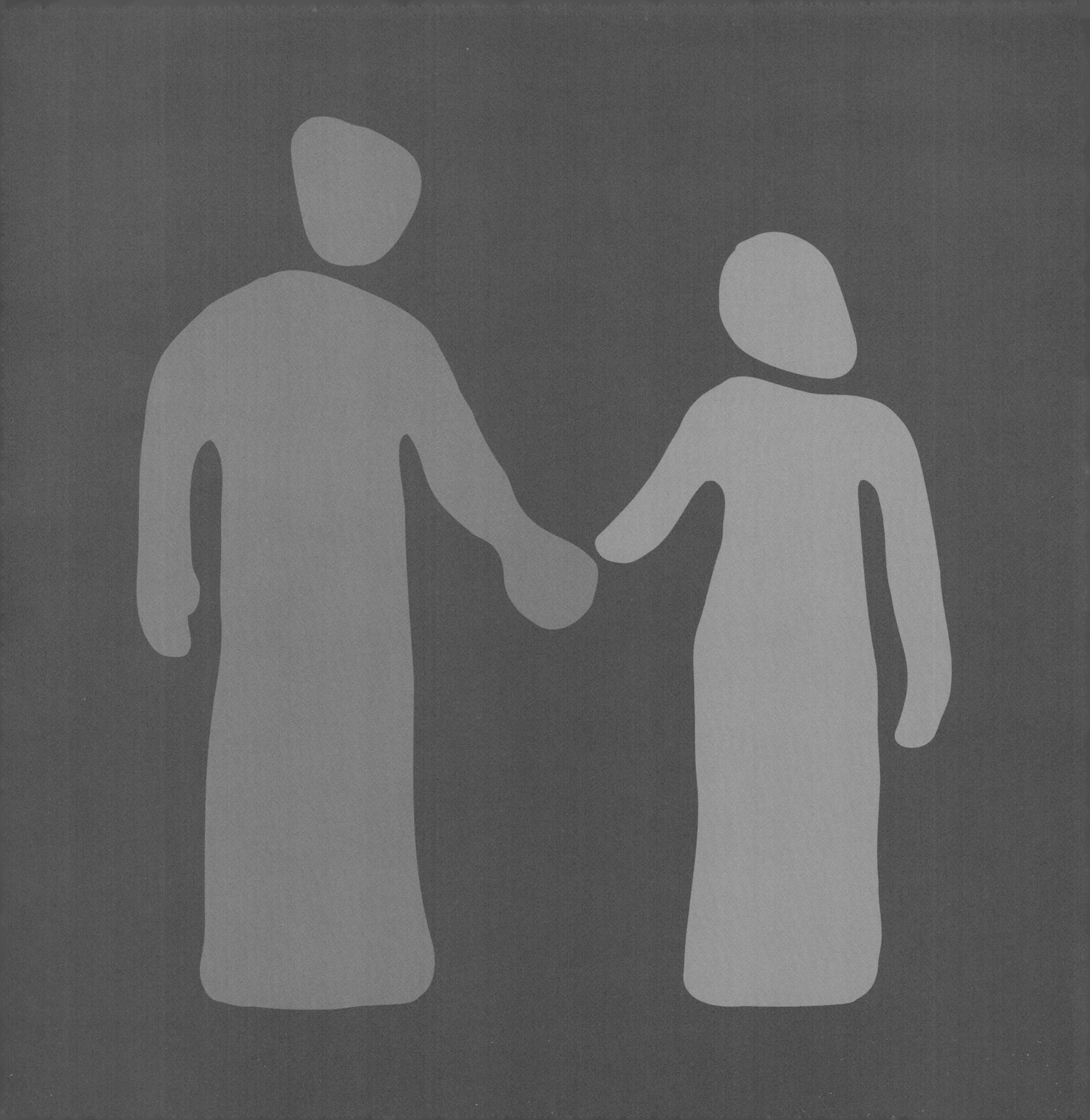

Friends 02

A life without friendship, however fleeting, is unimaginable. This probably tells you how important friends are.

All friendships are different. The motivation for friendships often varies depending on our needs at the time but ultimately a friendship, nurtured and worked at, is the greatest treasure we can carry around.

Ask yourself 'Why am I friends with this person?' and seek the truth. The answer will likely reveal an insight into your wellbeing and needs.

Friendships with family or otherwise, when everything else has been stripped away, are the basic core of everything rewarding and valuable in our lives. For most people, most of the time, experiences shared are **the golden moments that make a life joyous.**

"The bird a nest, the spider a web, man friendship." William Blake

"Friends can help each other. A true friend is someone who lets you have total freedom to be yourself - and especially to feel. Or, not feel. Whatever you happen to be feeling at the moment is fine with them. That's what real love amounts to - letting a person be what he really is." Jim Morrison

"Walking with a friend in the dark is better than walking alone in the light." Helen Keller

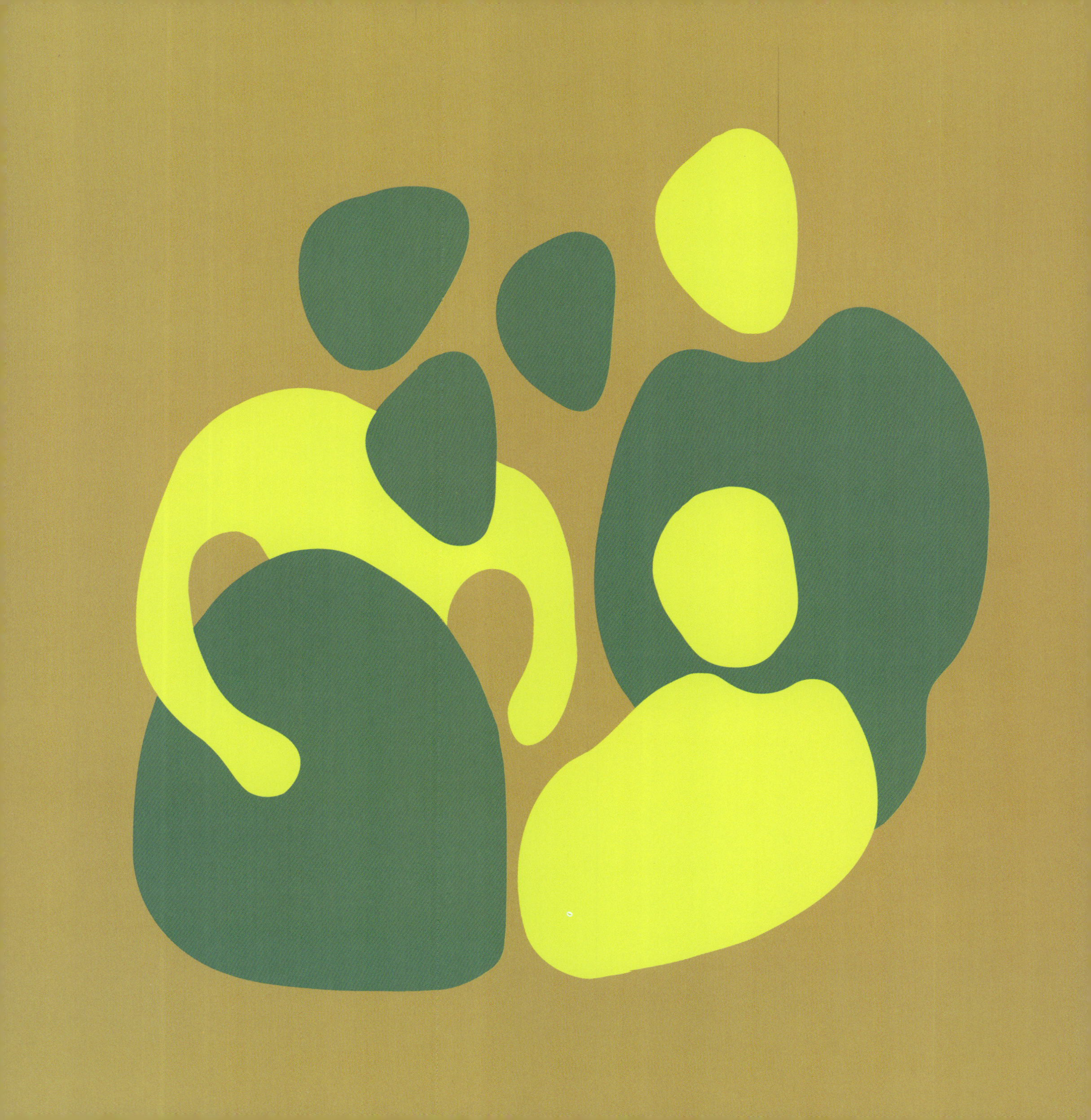

Family 03

Everything can be taught and passed on from parents. These lessons are different for all of us. It is important for everyone to find their own voice.

A family unit, if built well, can offer a great harbour for mental and physical rest, a sanctuary for learning about everything in the wider world and an early, safe place for examining relationships before embarking on the more turbulent seas of independence.

Next time you have to express an opinion on an important matter, ask yourself: Is this opinion mine? How much of it comes from my parents' and how much of it comes from my peer group? **What do I really believe?**

Understanding parental influences, their beliefs and values, and separating them from your own, is critical for building your independence and personal strength of wellbeing.

"The bond that links your true family is not one of blood, but of respect and joy in each other's life." Richard Bach

"In every conceivable manner, the family is link to our past, bridge to our future." Alex Haley

"Family is the most important thing in the world." Princess Diana

"The family is the nucleus of civilization." Will Durant

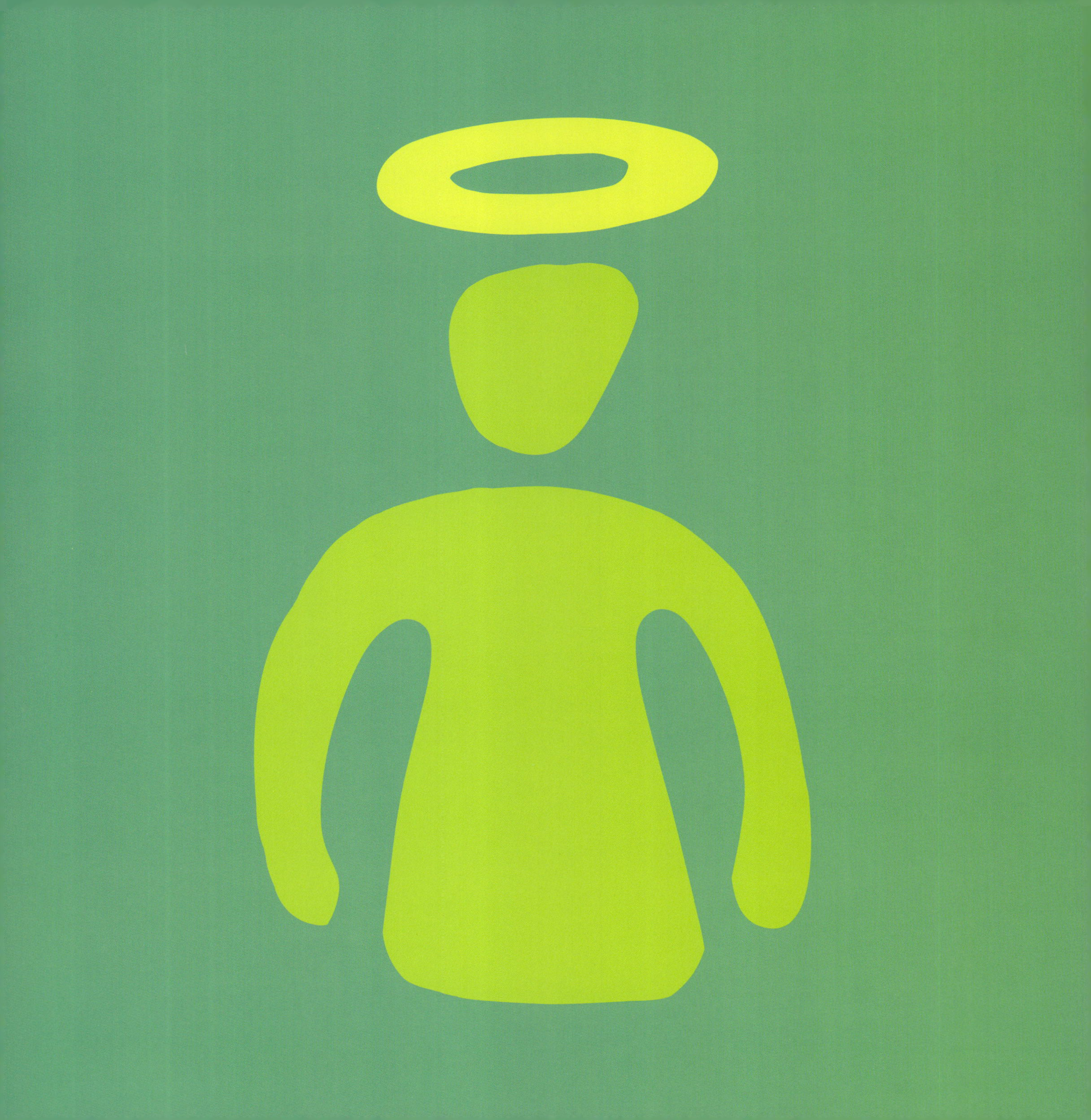

Honesty 04

Honesty with yourself is as important as it is with others. Anything less than the truth, when dealing with yourself and with others leads to a longer journey.

Concealing the truth or hiding the reality may offer an elastoplast or shortcut to short term gains, but for a solid foundation of belief in yourself and a wellbeing happiness, it is a better long term strategy to be **truthful with yourself**.

The question to ask and keep asking is one of the hardest - what is the truth of this? Is this really how this is? By learning to ask this simple but powerful question you are on a longer, but ultimately more rewarding, path to a fuller life.

The benefits of dealing honestly and openly with others, means they can learn to trust you more quickly, more people will want to spend time with you and ultimately perhaps share more experiences and a fuller life. Why waste your time spending more energy than you need to. Life is short.

"All truth passes through three stages. First, it is ridiculed. Second, it is violently opposed. Third, it is accepted as being self-evident."
Arthur Schopenhauer

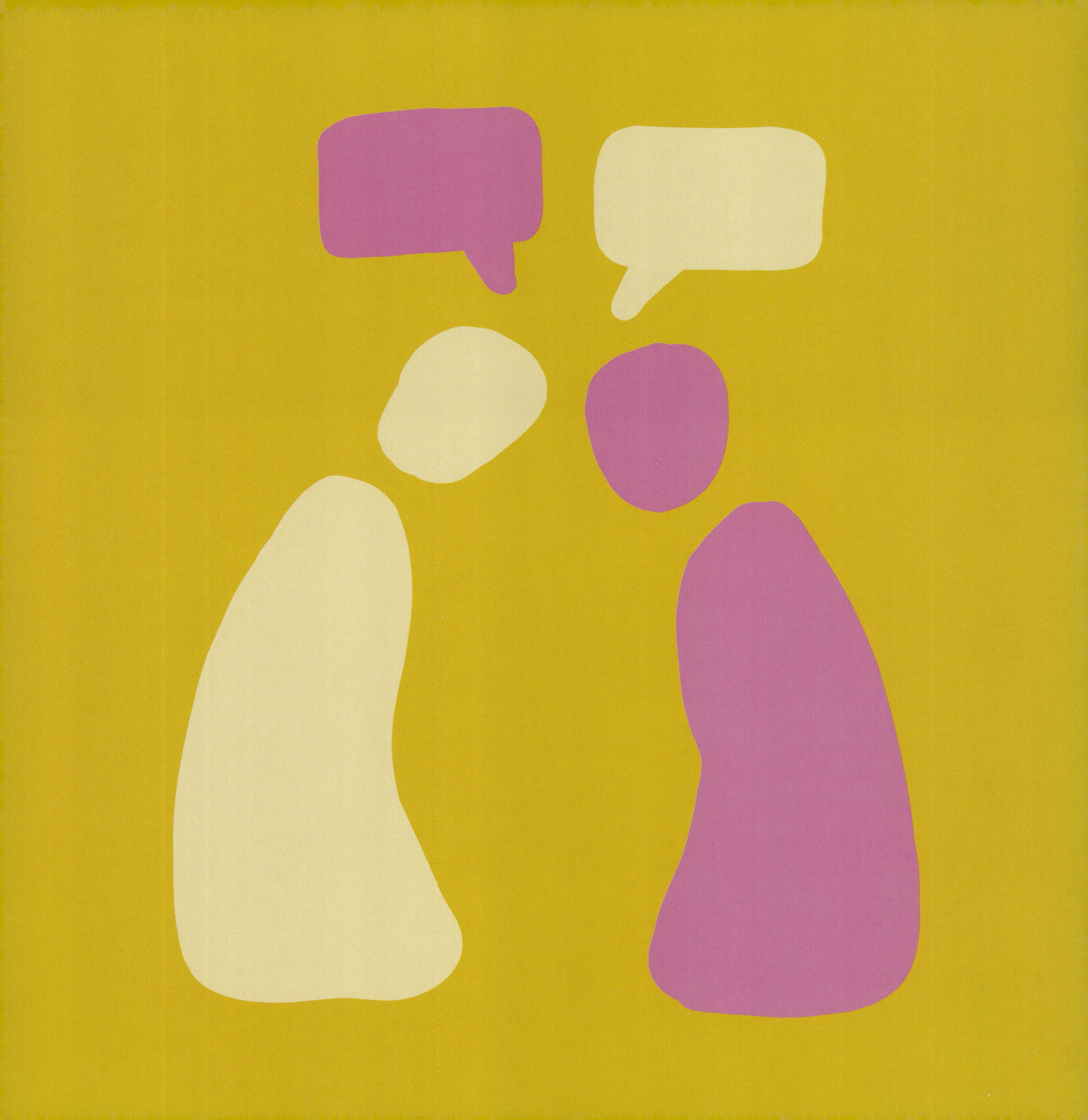

Talk 05

Good communication is at the heart of achieving harmony in relationships. Listening, looking and adjusting responses carefully in a conversation reveals truths.

Communication is **a two way process** you talk and you listen. It is important to actually hear and understand what is being said and they are often different things. To listen well is to observe and understand the other person's body language, emotions and verbal tone as much as the words they speak.

Ask yourself after a conversation 'Have I taken enough time to listen to, and have I really understood, what is actually being said?' Try to never assume anything, always ask 'Is this the truth of what I am being told'.

Practising listening and clearly and truthfully communicating well with others, will undoubtedly strengthen bonds and broaden your friendships. It makes sense that the more effectively you can do this, the more effective your personal growth and in turn your general feeling of wellbeing.

"Any problem, big or small, within a family, always seems to start with bad communication. Someone isn't listening." Emma Thompson

"To effectively communicate, we must realize that we are all different in the way we perceive the world and use this understanding as a guide to our communication with others." Tony Robbins

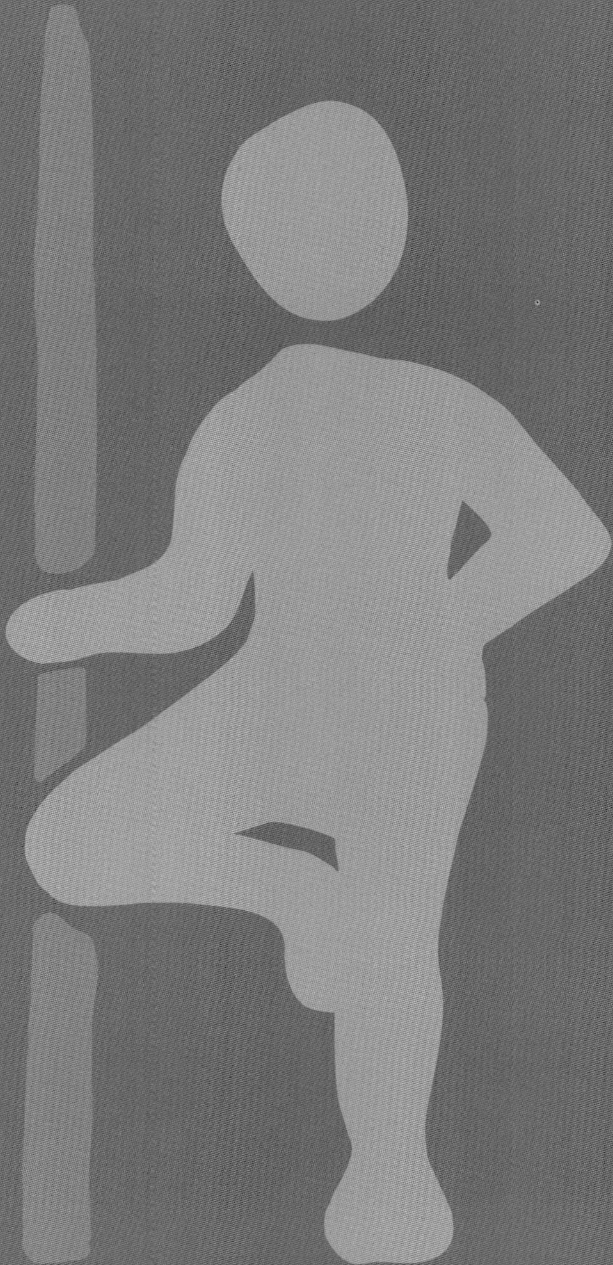

Tribe 06

Belonging to a tribe or community fills a primitive need to be a part of fellow humankind.

Tribes are a community that usually share your beliefs and values, a group of like-minded individuals. It is as important to belong and learn from the time spent in these groups as it is to spend time alone and learning about yourself. Ultimately, we function more strongly when we have adopted individual responsibility for ourselves.

Ask yourself What do I love doing? Is there a way of sharing this? Try setting yourself a goal of trying out new groups with an open-minded approach that embraces the possibility of **learning more about yourself through interaction** and shared experience with others.

If the goal is to belong, then by definition it is probably important to find a place in a tribe. The benefits will be a warmth if it shares your views and a growth if it challenges your opinions.

"There is as much to be gained from belonging to a tribe, seeing the reflection of yourself, learning to develop long, lasting and meaningful bonds with others, as there is to be gained by investigation of your relationship with yourself." Anon.

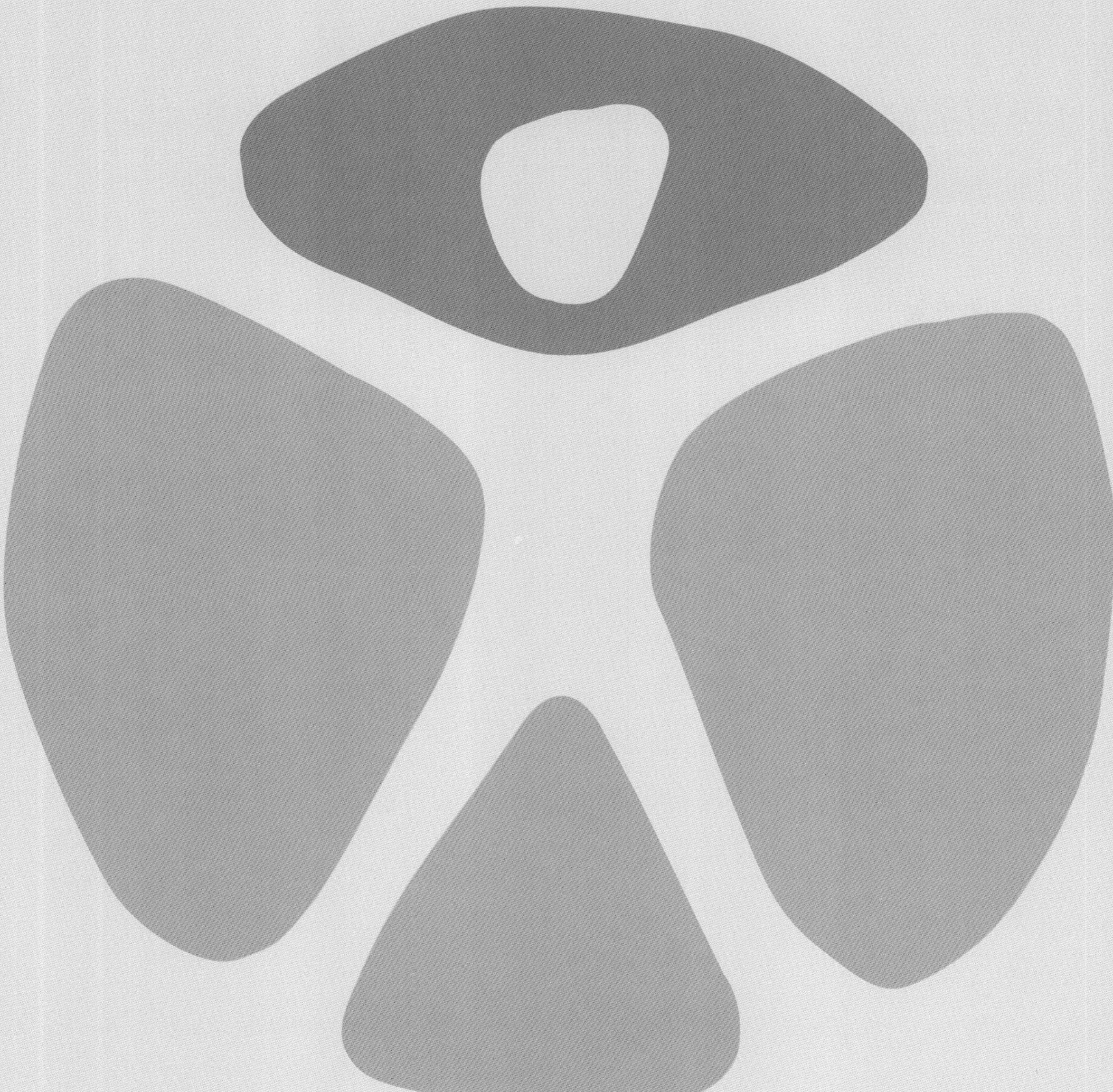

Belonging 07

The ties that bind. Feeling you belong to others, with all its positive aspects, can leave a feeling of good on the inside, adding significantly to your bank of wellbeing.

Feeling alone, feelings of loneliness or isolation are amongst the most common of human emotions reported. There are tendencies to exaggerate these feelings inwardly and sometimes your outward behaviour exacerbates the feelings, which in turn can create a problem which was originally entirely in your head.

Exercise: Try finding the **fun things you enjoy doing** and join a club or community project that enjoys doing the same activity.

Love and belonging are the most essential basics of human needs. We are hard-wired, if you believe we are pack animals, to belong to the group. The positive and reinforced feelings of being a part of something bigger than you are, arguably, is a very primitive need.

"A deep sense of love and belonging is an irreducible need of all people."
Brene Brown

"You cannot change any society unless you take responsibility for it, unless you see yourself as belonging to it and responsible for changing it."
Grace Lee Boggs

"You are not alone. This is probably one of the most reassuring sentiments we can ever hear."

"At the end of the day, it's the people around us who build our happiest moments."

1 Summary

Being a part of something, laughing, crying and sharing life with all its emotions with others is part of our pack instinct.

We are all different, we all have different needs and this will vary through our lives, but one thing is certain, we all need each other to some extent or the other, if only to go for a walk or to the coffee shop with someone.

We need to talk, we need friends who listen, care and watch our backs, we need to feel we are part of humankind with all its faults and foibles. Our flaws make us the characters we are.

We are wonderfully humourously, sentimentally bonkers and this universal club of human-kind can do amazing things... but only together.

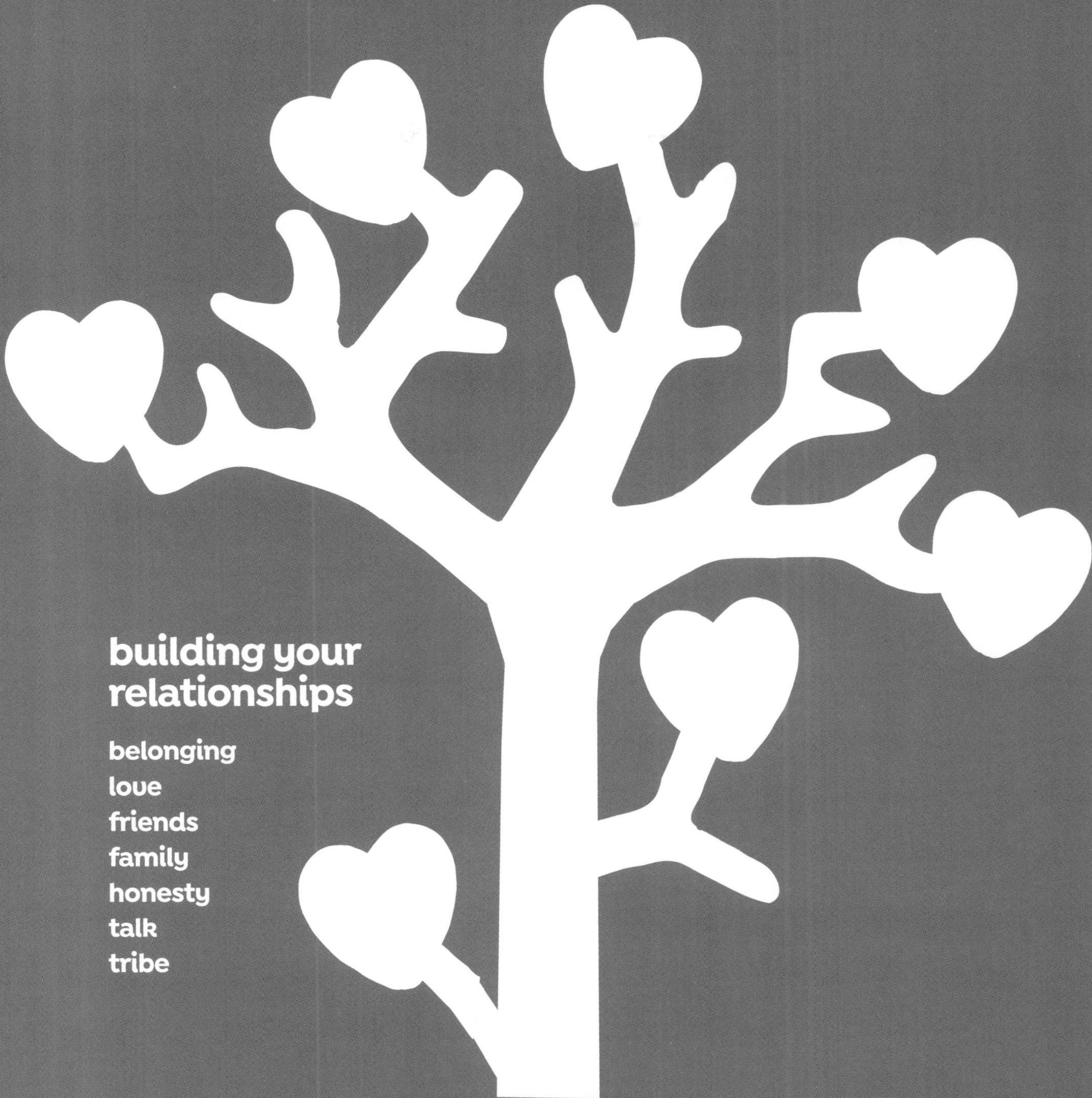

building your relationships

belonging
love
friends
family
honesty
talk
tribe

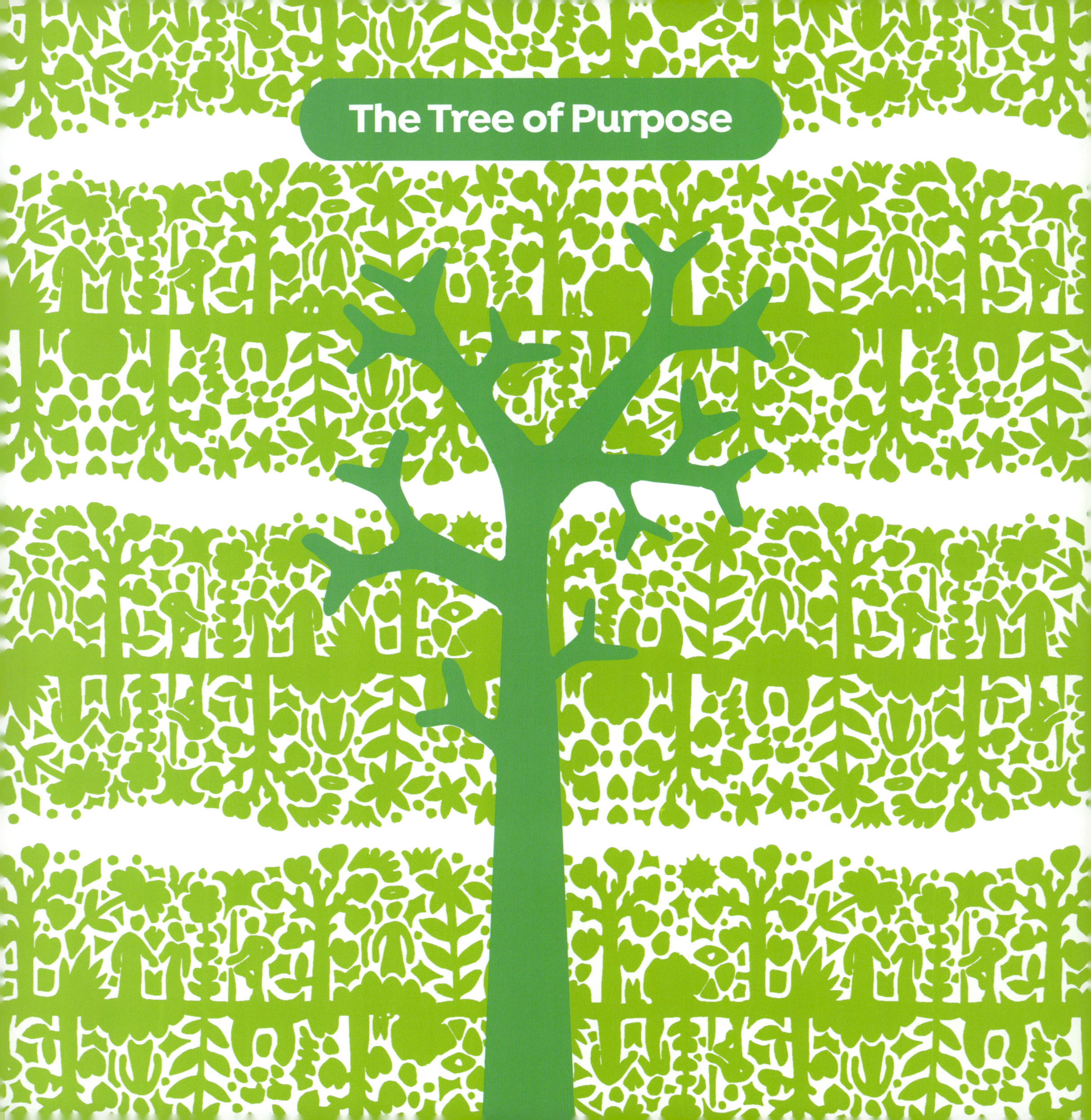
The Tree of Purpose

2

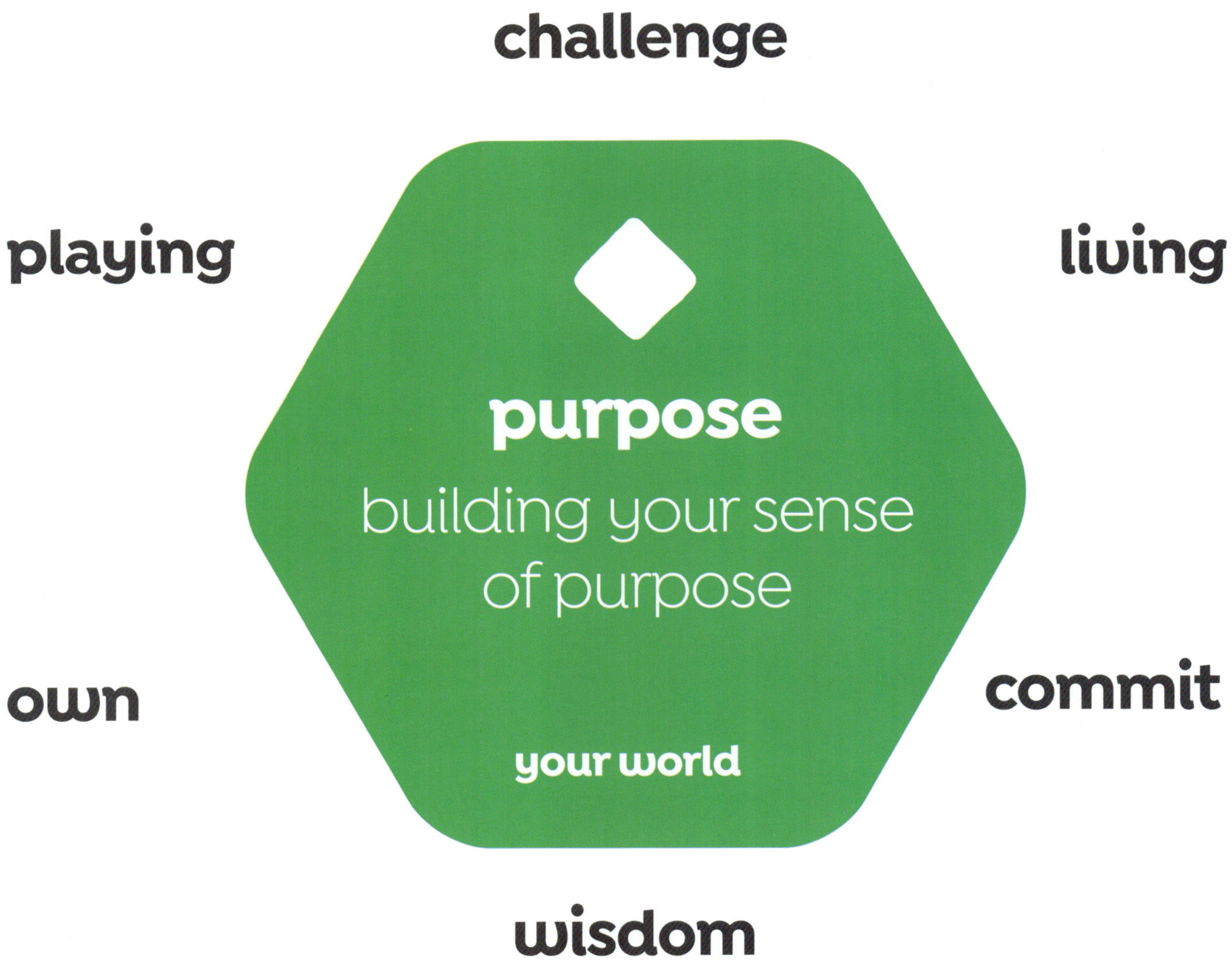
challenge
playing
living
purpose
building your sense of purpose
own
commit
your world
wisdom

2 Your World

The second tree in the Magic Forest of wellbeing is the tree of purpose, and it is all about finding your place in this world.

The following keywords will help you build your sense of purpose by questioning and understanding how you choose to live, play, and commit to challenges. The words of this tree help you ask the questions you need to ask to develop a better and more solid wellbeing. Finding your own place in the world will help you find your own personal wisdom and the responsibility of owning your life.

The following questions, quotes and insights are a summary of the essential elements to help you start building your understanding of, and finding your place in, the world one action or one deed at a time.

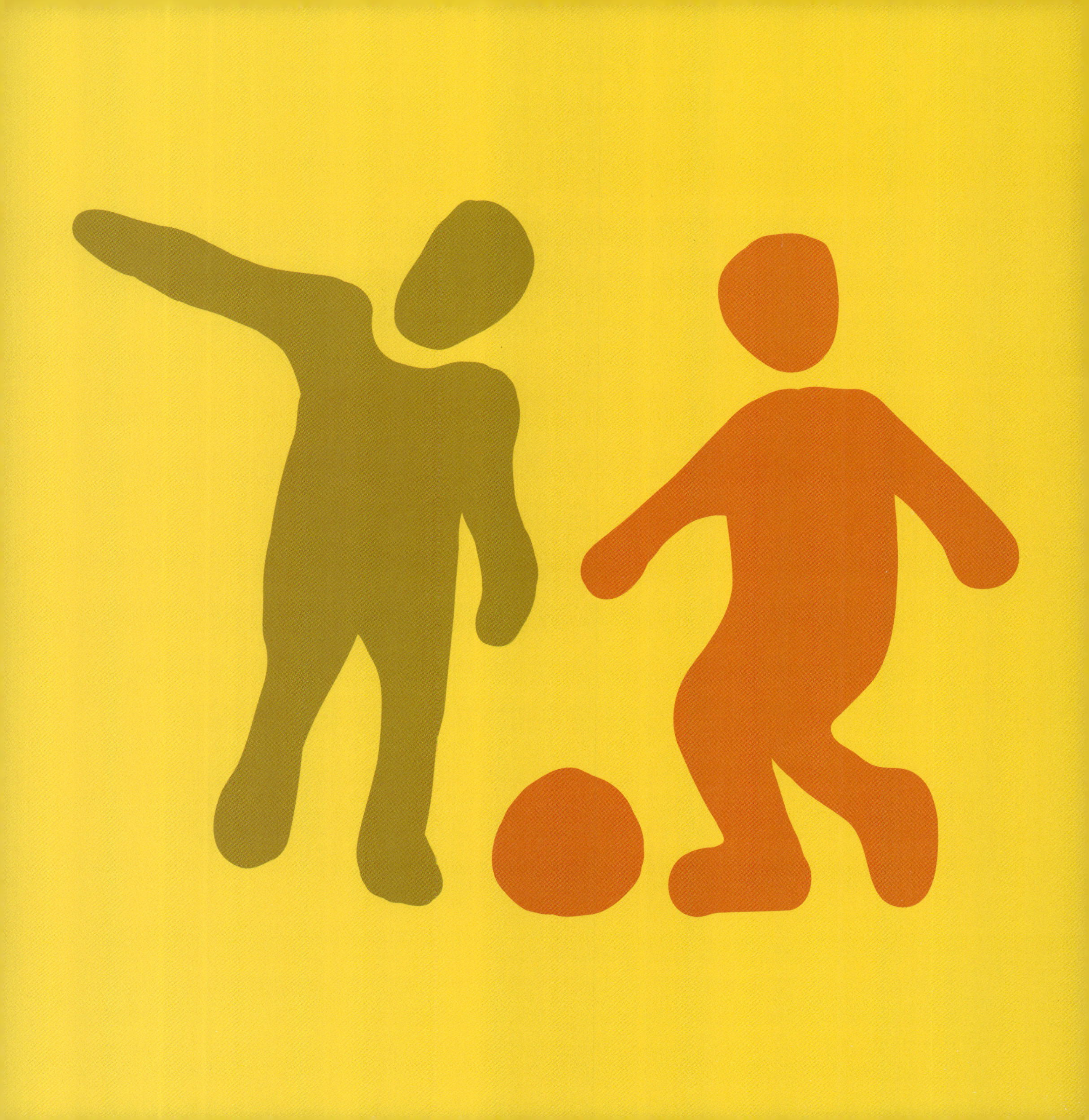

Playing 08

A life full of joy and laughter, a childlike love of new things and the curiosity to explore them will yield a rich and full life.

Aiming for the goal of a childlike curiosity can be an artistic ambition, but the same curiosity enrichens your life and those around you across all the arts from dancing, singing, painting, writing and any form where you can express yourself.

Ask yourself what is stopping me from doing something. Get deeply honest about what you love doing and ask 'Why can't I do that?'

Finding and building your best self for a good life means exploring several paths, it is **a creative process** requiring a mind open to the possibilities of new things. Trying new things, embracing these moments adds to your bank of wellbeing and the challenge can teach you things about yourself.

"Without creativity, there would be no progress, and we would be forever repeating the same patterns." Edward de Bono

"We don't stop playing because we grow old; we grow old because we stop playing." George Bernard Shaw

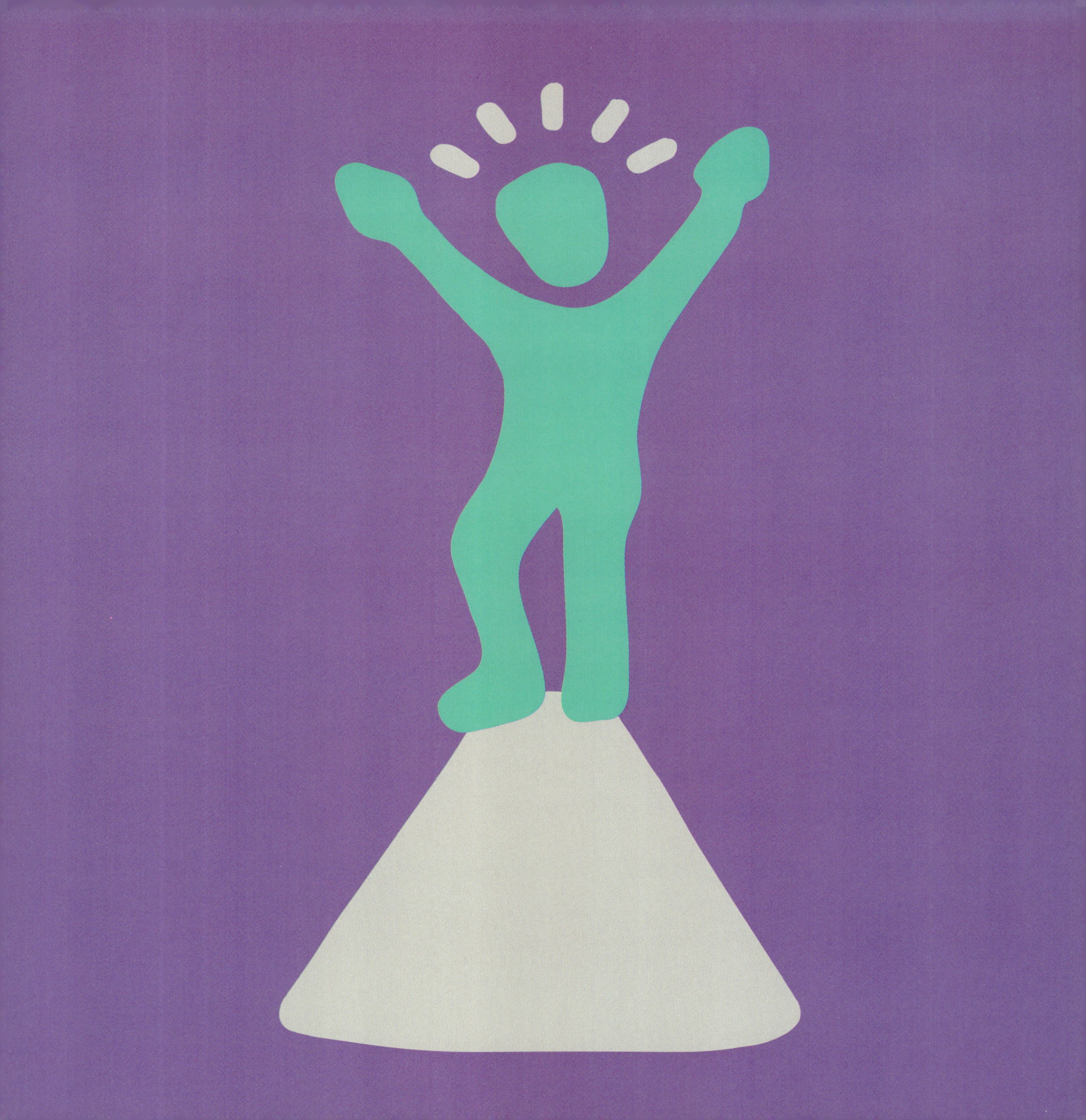

Living

09

Loving what you do for a living and living your life to the fullest will ensure a life with no regrets later on. Make it count... boom!

The more you do, the more experiences you have. **Experiences pretty much define your life**. After that it's about the quality and nature of the experience, and all the nuanced detail of whether it's adding to you in the way you would wish or otherwise.

Who do you believe has lived the fullest life and serves as a great example? Ask yourself the question, 'Why do I admire them so much?' It will probably reveal great insights into your own life and lifestyle. Note: Making heroes of personalities is often disappointing. Perhaps you could be your own hero?

Feeling truly alive and vital can come as a result of an extreme situation where your life is in danger. Extreme sports can offer this life affirmation, but I cannot recommend this in these notes.

"The purpose of life is to live it, to taste experience to the utmost, to reach out eagerly and without fear for newer and richer experience." Eleanor Roosevelt

"You are what you do, not what you say you do." Carl Jung

"Enjoy the little things in life, for one day you may look back and realise they were the big things." Robert Bault

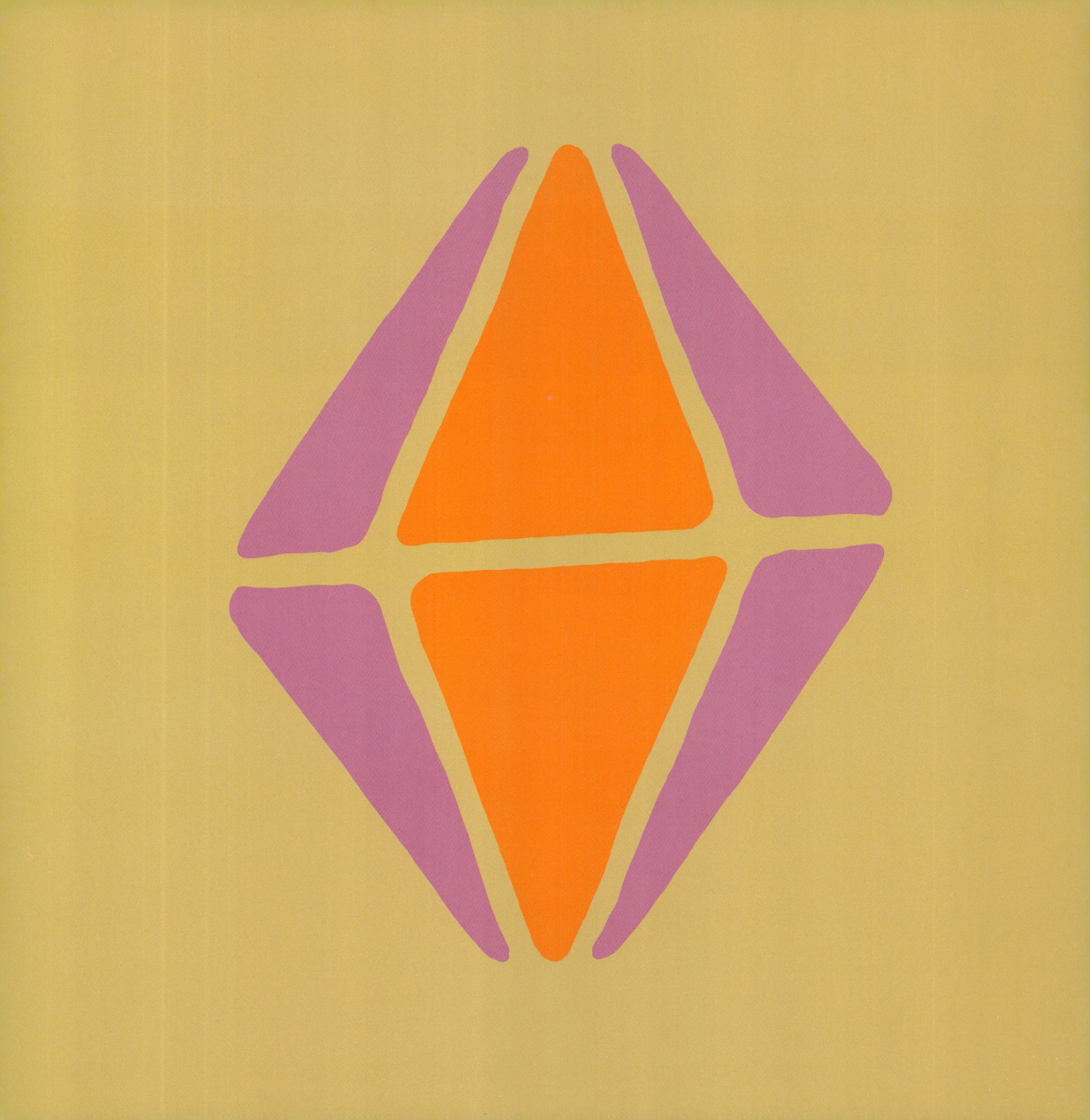

Wisdom 10

The quality of good judgement is learning from experience, continually asking questions, and finding your own way of understanding the answers.

Wisdom is defined as the quality of having **experience, knowledge, and good judgement.** A big part of being confident in your own decisions is knowing you can make mistakes. Doing your best to consider all aspects and potential outcomes, of any decision on a path, are very much a part of the process that takes you to a planned destination such as your strong wellbeing.

Think about your future self, what are they like or what would you like them to be like and factor this into your decision. Ask yourself, "What would my future me do in this situation?"

Wise and considered decisions are the bedrock of a good life. The better the decisions you make the greater the quality of life you will ultimately have.

"A society grows great when old men plant trees whose shade they know they shall never sit in." Greek Proverb

"Wise men talk because they have something to say; Fools, because they have to say something" Plato

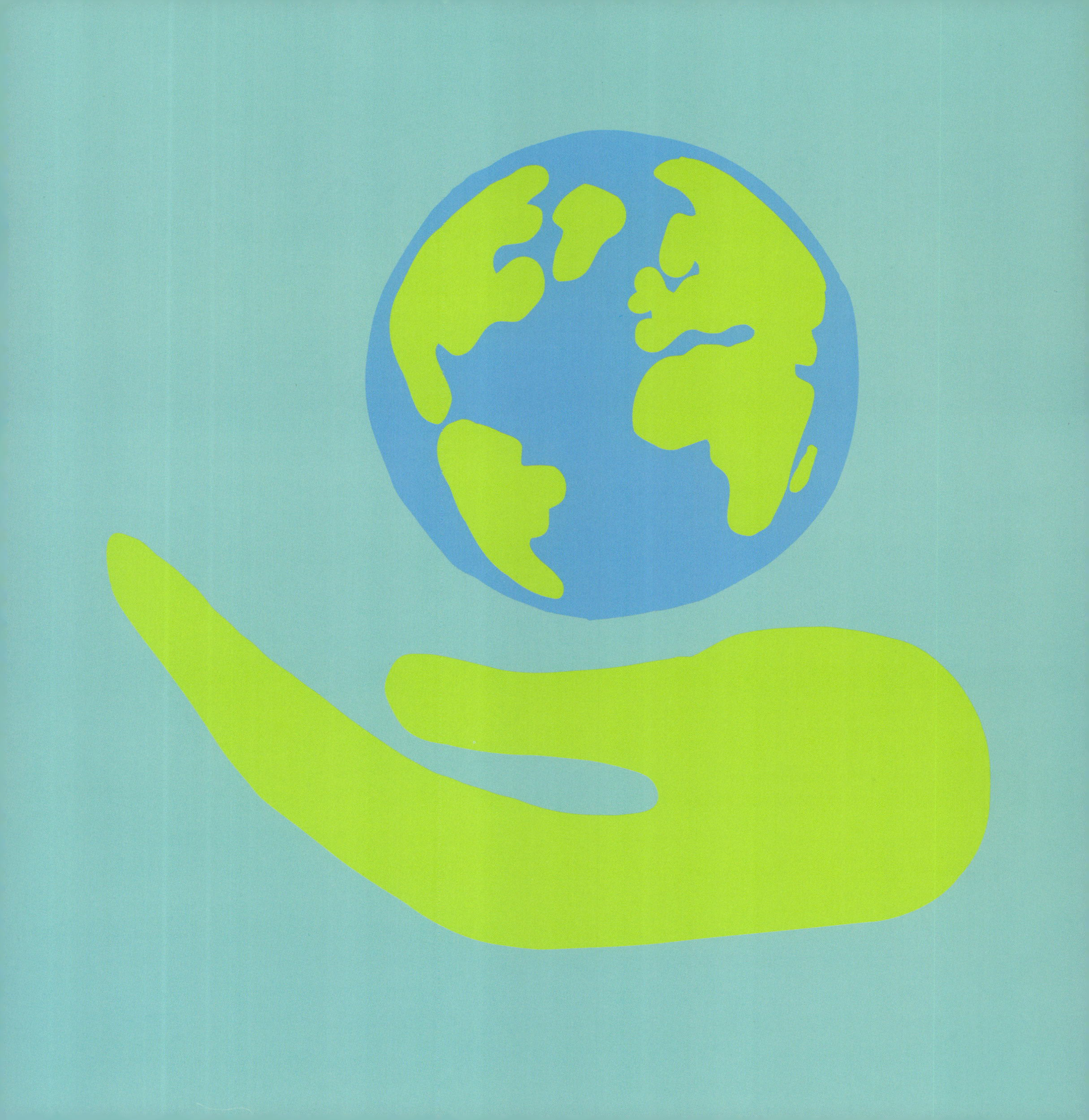

◆ Own 11

Taking responsibility for your own life is a key developmental milestone. Owning your own life and taking responsibility for others can be the best of being human.

A responsible lifestyle can add meaning as well as purpose to your life. Passing the milestone in your life when you realise and accept your responsibilities not only defines you but is an unforgettable moment in your life, **a rite of passage** to being all human.

Ask yourself, 'What is the difference between a child and an adult and when did I become an adult? The difference is usually responsibility at some point in our lives.

The self-respect you earn for yourself, and earn from others, for owning your own decisions, taking full responsibility for your life and those under your wing, feels good. Extending this responsibility and 'giving a care' beyond immediate family to friends, colleagues, and the world in general, when balanced, can feel even better. Add to this the importance as a species of collective responsibility for our planet and it all becomes seriously important.

"A nation is formed by the willingness of each of us to share in the responsibility for upholding the common good." Barbara Jordan

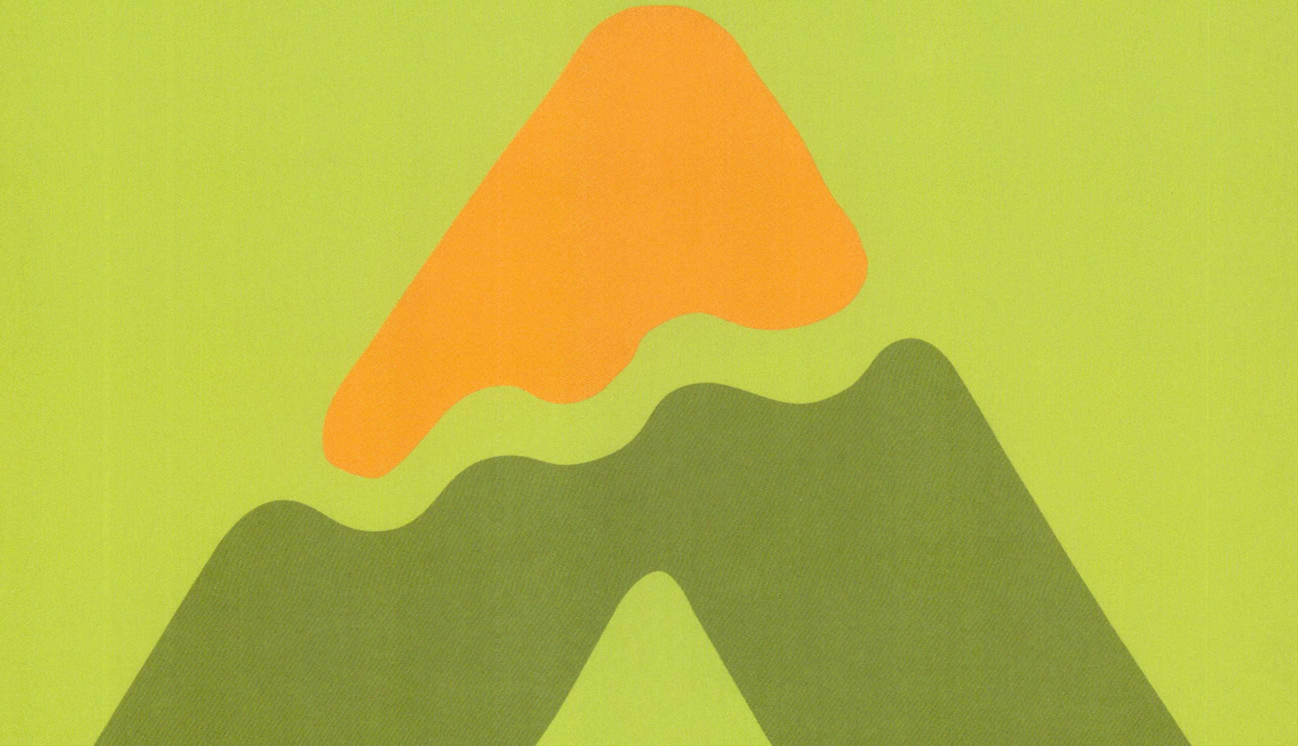

Challenge 12

Getting out of your comfort zone and taking up a challenge will develop skills that stay with you and build you forever.

To succeed in any goal or challenge, you will a particular skill set for the task, then commitment. focus, persistence, and resilience probably in that order. **Setting goals is important**, as with planning, failing to plan will probably ensure you never reach your goal.

In order to maximise your chances of reaching your goal it is always worth asking 'How can I break down my goal into a series of smaller achievable steps?'

By stretching yourself and undertaking a challenge you will stretch the boundaries of what you know about yourself. The knowledge of **what you can and can't do, will give you a greater confidence** in yourself and a greater sense of overall wellbeing.
Understanding and minimising stress is important for facing a challenge. Stress is, for the most part, simply the difference between what you perceive or think you can do and what you actually can do. Learning this is a great starting point to taking on a challenge.

"We don't plan to fail, we simply fail to plan. Having no plan will certainly ensure you get to one place - nowhere." Anon.

100%

Commit 13

Commitment is an essential step for any goal. It opens doors and yields surprising results, with hidden rewards you have no idea about until you walk into them.

Commitment to your life decisions will add to your sense of purpose and show you the way. Even if you make some wrong decisions, the likelihood is **failure will teach you a great deal.**

Exercise: Choose one of your goals and knowing that failure will teach you a great deal, try asking yourself 'Am I prepared to accept the outcome and responsibility of what happens if I fail to reach this goal?'

Undertaking a goal and committing to it to the end will require both hard work and doing things you are uncomfortable with such as sacrifice, but it will be fulfilling in the end. It will teach you about yourself and you will certainly grow as a person. The commitment is often seen as the first step, but every step will require **commitment coupled to hard and smart work** in order to achieve success.

"Once you have commitment, you need the discipline and hard work to get you there." Haile Gebrselassie

"Commitment transforms a promise into reality" Abraham Lincoln

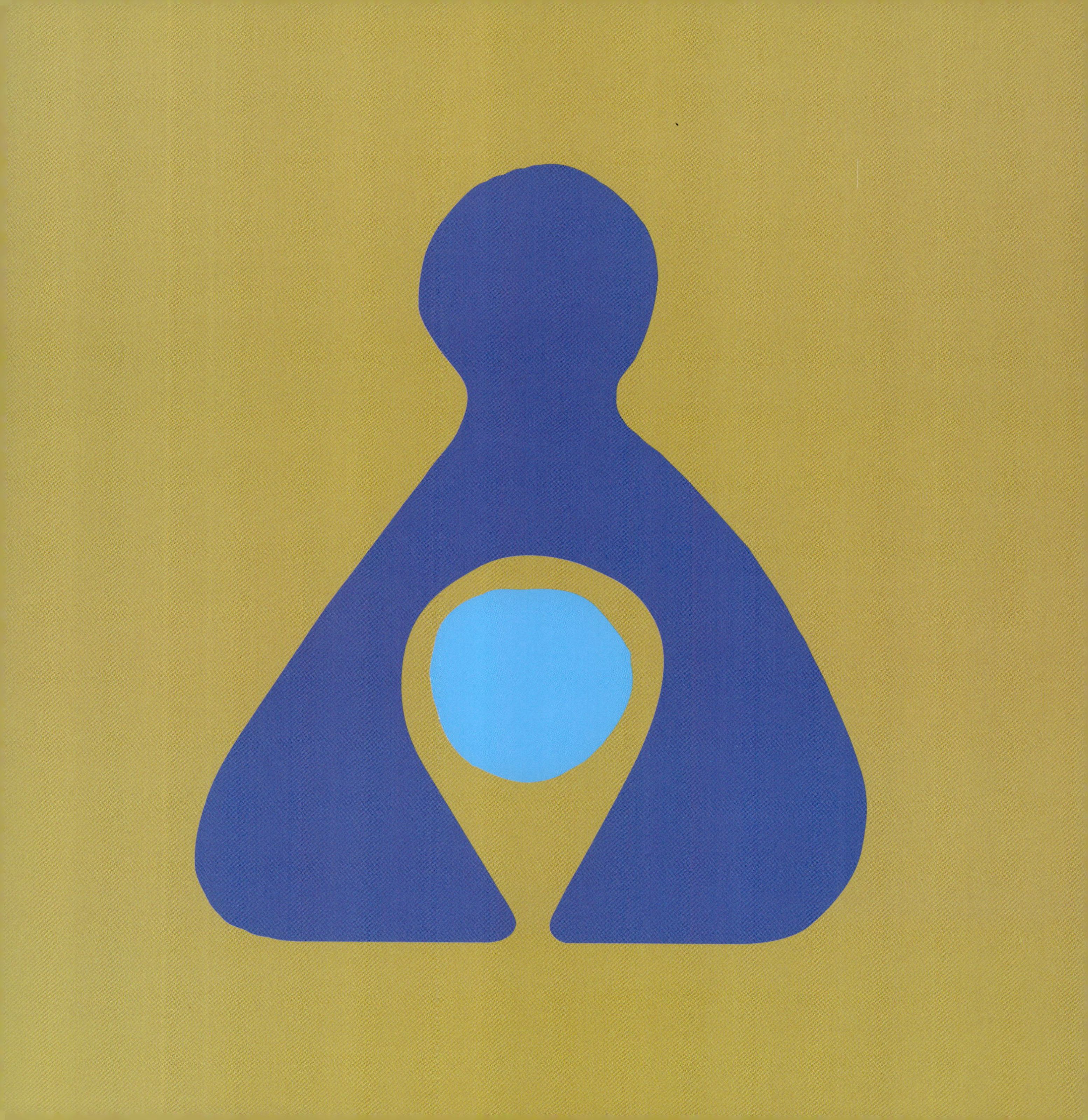

Purpose 14

Your sense of purpose in the world can be simply defined as the reasons you get out of bed in the morning.

The meaning of your life can be defined as your personal choice of purpose. Heavy philosophical argument taken further may simply cloud your decision and potentially waste lots of valuable time that could be spent doing the things you love.

Finding your purpose may not be easy. But it will certainly be a combination of the **things you love to do**. Ask yourself 'Which jobs seem to make time fly by and what do I really love doing?'

The process of asking what you love doing and reasoning why you love doing it may take time. It may take a lifetime and the answer may have been under your nose all along, but when you eventually know it feels great. However simple, it is **your reason**, it is very personal and it can put a spring in your step if you are still bendy enough by the time you find out what it is.

"The mystery of human existence lies not in just staying alive, but in finding something to live for." Fyodor Dostoyevsky

"The purpose of life is a life of purpose" Robert Byrne.

"Until you have searched with honesty to know a little more about yourself, it is unlikely you will find the greatest treasure of all... doing what you love."

“Avoid the cliché – spending money we don’t have, to buy things we don’t need, to impress people we don’t like.”

2 Summary

Finding your place in a world of eight billion people is no easy task. The start and end point is to do what you love doing.

In choosing what we do with our lives we often end up going down several wrong roads.

One of the greatest flaws in our thinking seems to be that we try and strengthen what we are weak at rather than playing to our strengths.

Generally speaking, if we do what we love we will be good at it, or at least get better quicker until those skills are both pleasurable and useful.

Keep asking questions about yourself and your passions. If you keep trying new things, you will probably find some really useful answers to your personal meaning of life.

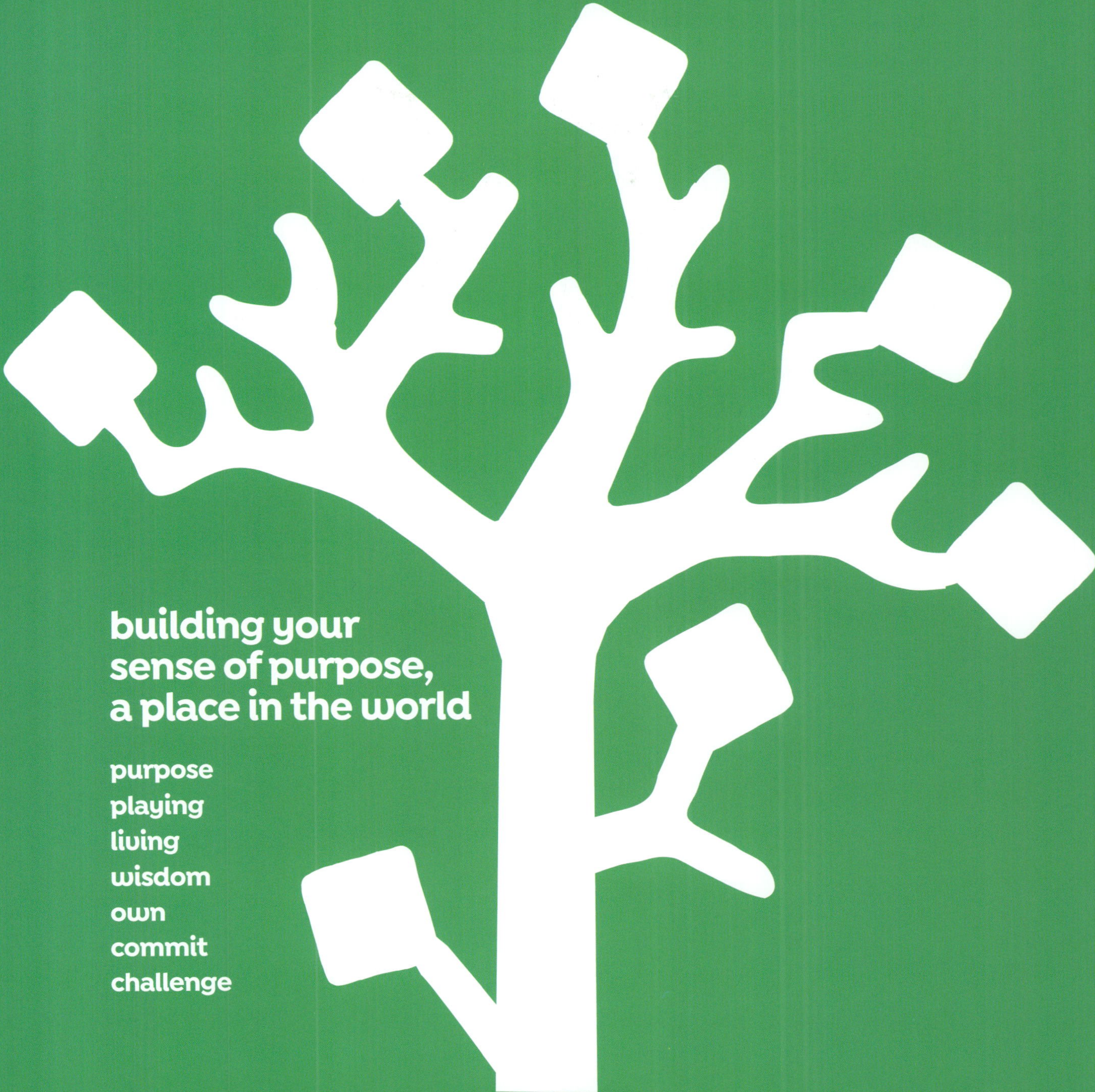

building your sense of purpose, a place in the world

purpose
playing
living
wisdom
own
commit
challenge

The Tree of Time

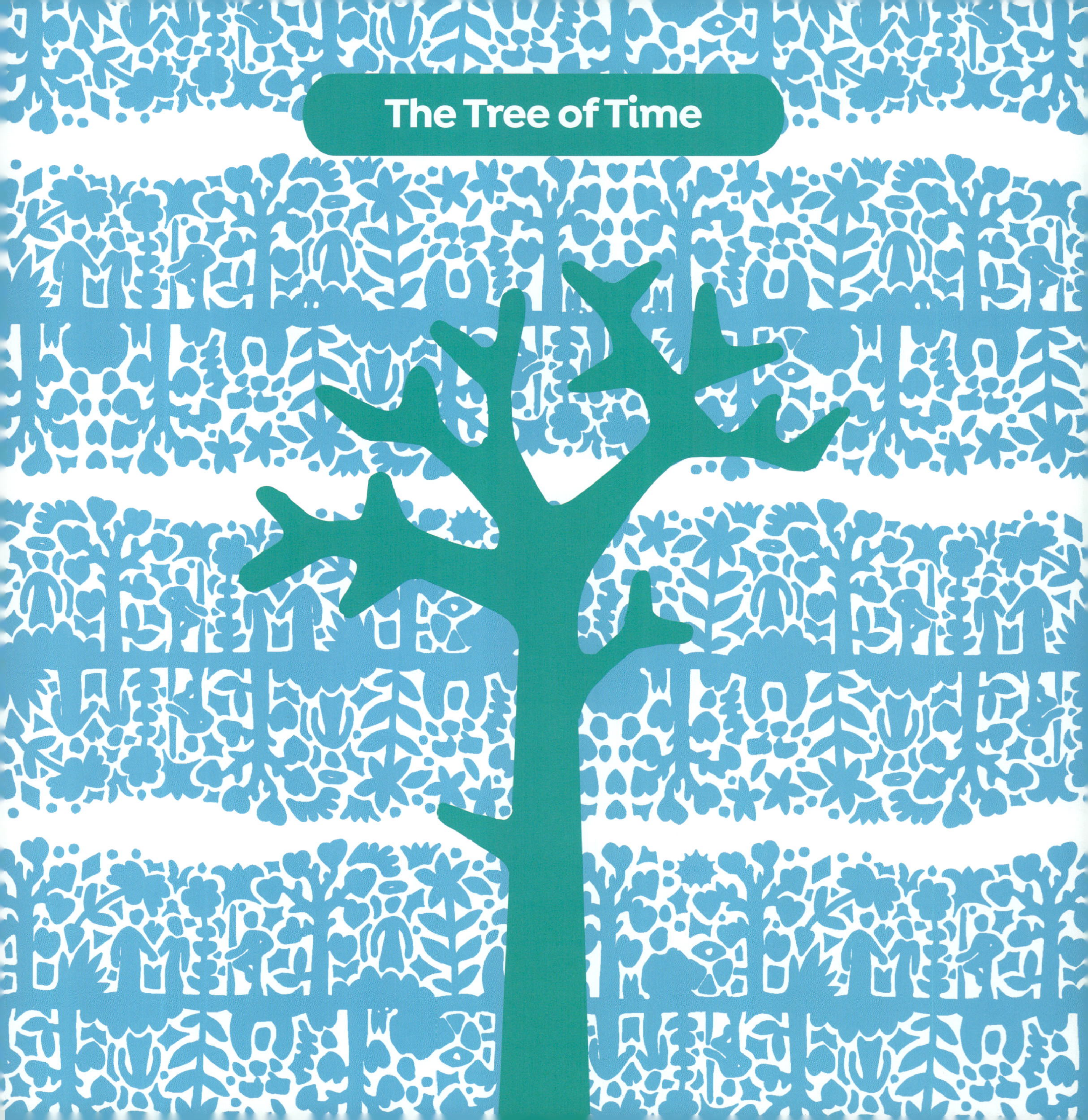

3

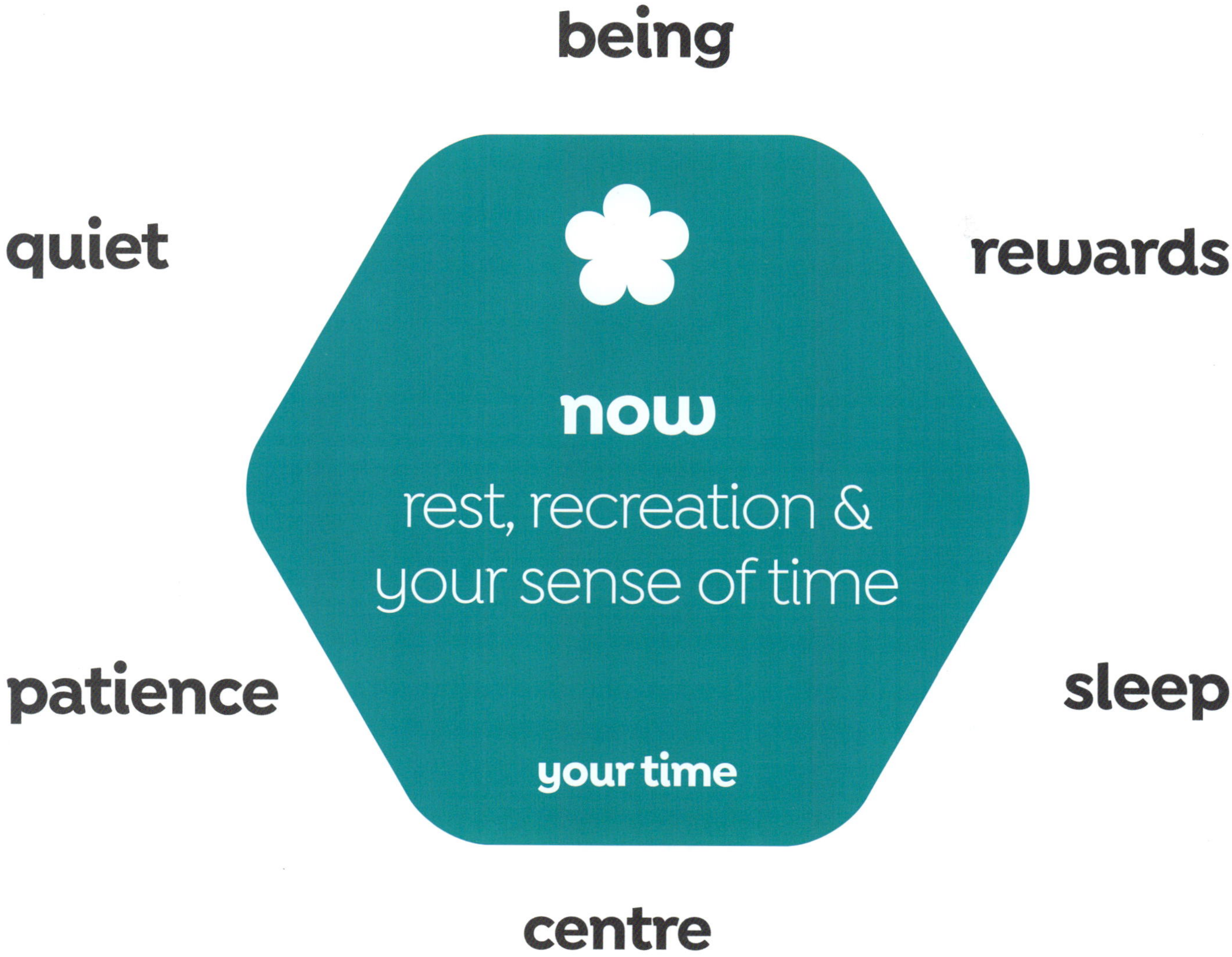

being
quiet
rewards
now
rest, recreation &
your sense of time
patience
sleep
your time
centre

3 Your Time

The third tree in the Magic Forest of wellbeing, the tree of time, is all about making the most of your sense of time.

The following keywords are about building your sense of time through living in the now, being present, focusing and centreing. These words help build an understanding of your need for quiet personal time, proper rest and recreation and the importance of sleep.

When you couple this with your motivations and rewards, you can attain a wonderful sense of slow and a calm inner place you can call upon for a more solid wellbeing.

The following questions, quotes and insights are a summary of essential elements to help you start understanding your own time, finding your sense of calm and inner peace.

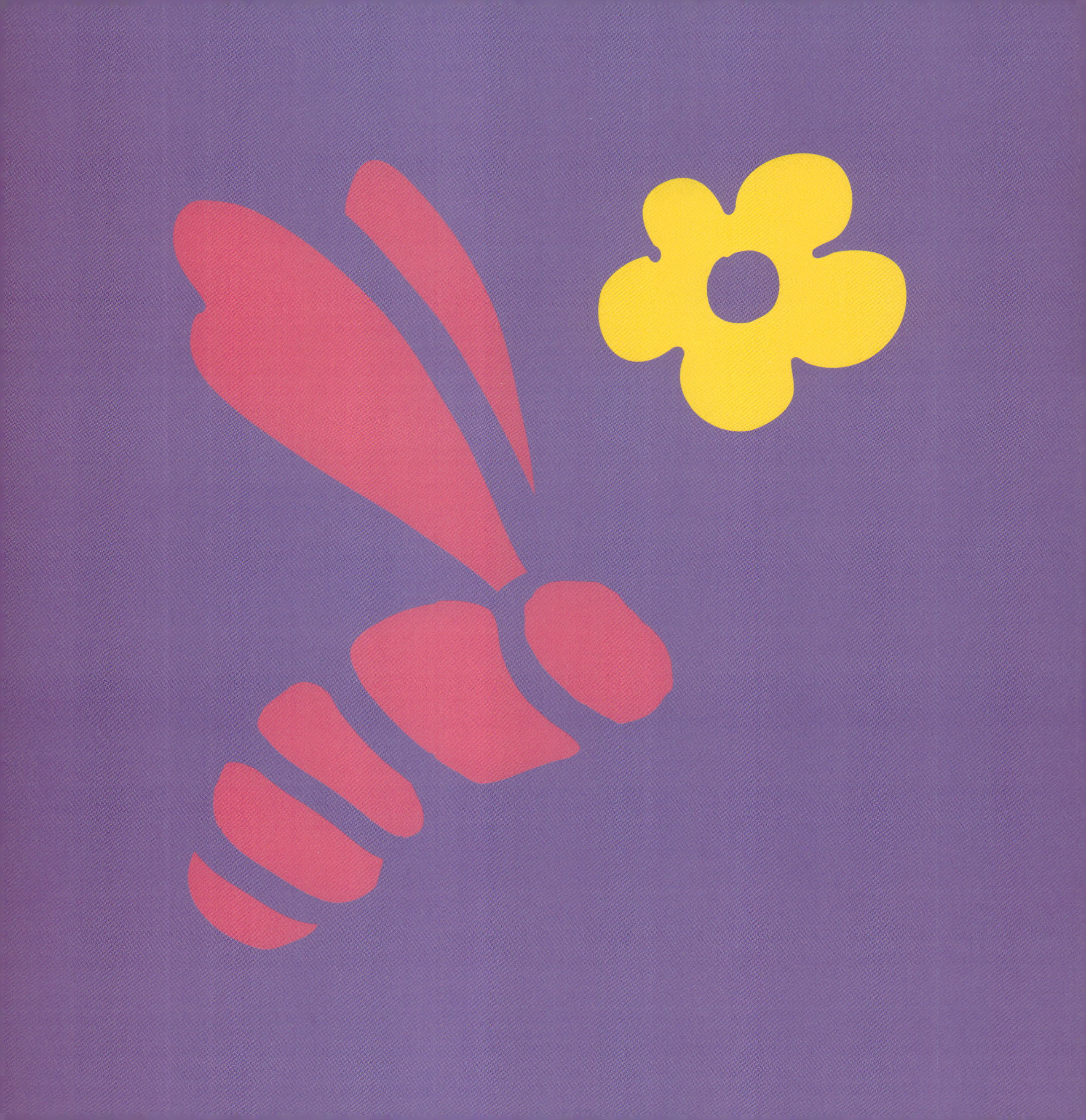

Be 15

Find the time to be in the space you are in, this will relax you. Learn to take the time to simply breathe and look around you.

Just being, just existing and creating some physical and mental space to free yourself. Just breathing, listening to the sound of silence, smelling the flowers, feeling your heart beat as you stride across a moor. **The simplest pleasures make the greatest experiences where time stands still**.

Next time you visit a park and you're feeling anxious about something, try an exercise for yourself. Take the time to stop, take a seat and focus on the nature that's going on around you. There is a whole lot more than is apparent at first. These minor discoveries will refresh you?

A pause in between the various tasks of the day can give you enough time to find a connection with the world out there. Feeling the great vastness of nature and the joy of all things alive can be in the smallest moment on the tiniest patch of green. Just look. The smallest lifts all add up to a greater whole.

"When the green woods laugh with the voice of joy, And the dimpling stream runs laughing by; When the air does laugh with our merry wit, And the green hill laughs with the noise of it."
William Blake

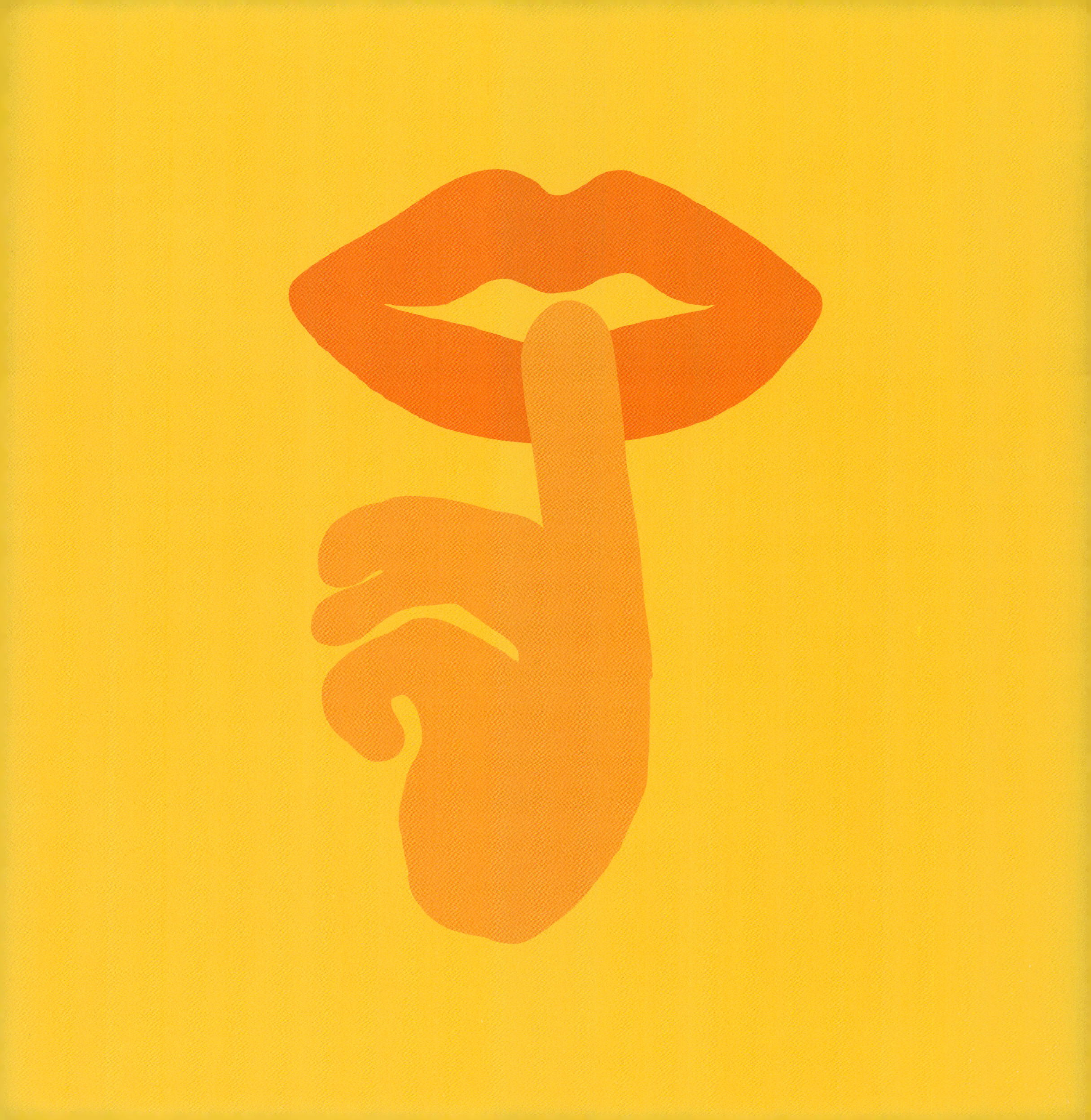

Quiet

16

Down time, me time free from the noise of the everyday, like the peace and quiet of nature, is a human essential for health.

Quiet, apart from the physical reality of external noise, is a freedom from the internal 'mind chatter' of daily thoughts. Exercise may purge much of this noise, but similarly certain good conversations and good sleep can create necessary space to clear the fog and ultimately perhaps make better life decisions.

An exercise to determine the difference between physical silence and an inner quiet might be to seek a quiet place when your head is full of anxieties and compare it to being in a busy room when you are full of peace and inner calm.

Quiet, especially the likes of the 'green quiet' of the countryside, provides a part of the mental and physical space necessary to process the day's activities and conversations properly. It will make way for **a clear head, improved concentration and general wellbeing** as the external and internal stress reduces.

"Only by going alone in silence, without baggage, can one truly get into the heart of the wilderness. All other travel is mere dust and hotels and baggage and chatter." John Muir

Centre 17

There is a calm place of peace, your centre, that is part of your rest and recreation time. Finding your own place, your centre, is bliss.

Returning to your inner calm, to the place in your mind where your heart slows, **your thoughts slow and you breathe easily** can be learnt. Your 'centre' is a balance point between the pull from many directions, where the day to day is put aside and your inner you is free to relax and enjoy happier thoughts. Finding this place, the process of centreing takes practise.

Exercise: Find a place in your mind where you were at ease, happy and content. Try to keep revisiting this place and see how more relaxed you can become each time you visit.

The health benefits of rest and recreation, of being calm and relaxed are seemingly obvious, but the hidden benefits of being in control of finding your place are less so. Learning to understand how to get to your meditative core, your centre, allows you to calm down from day-to-day stresses on demand. This knowledge and technique can provide **great mental and physical ease**.

"I have begun to think of life as a series of ripples widening out from an original centre." Seamus Heaney

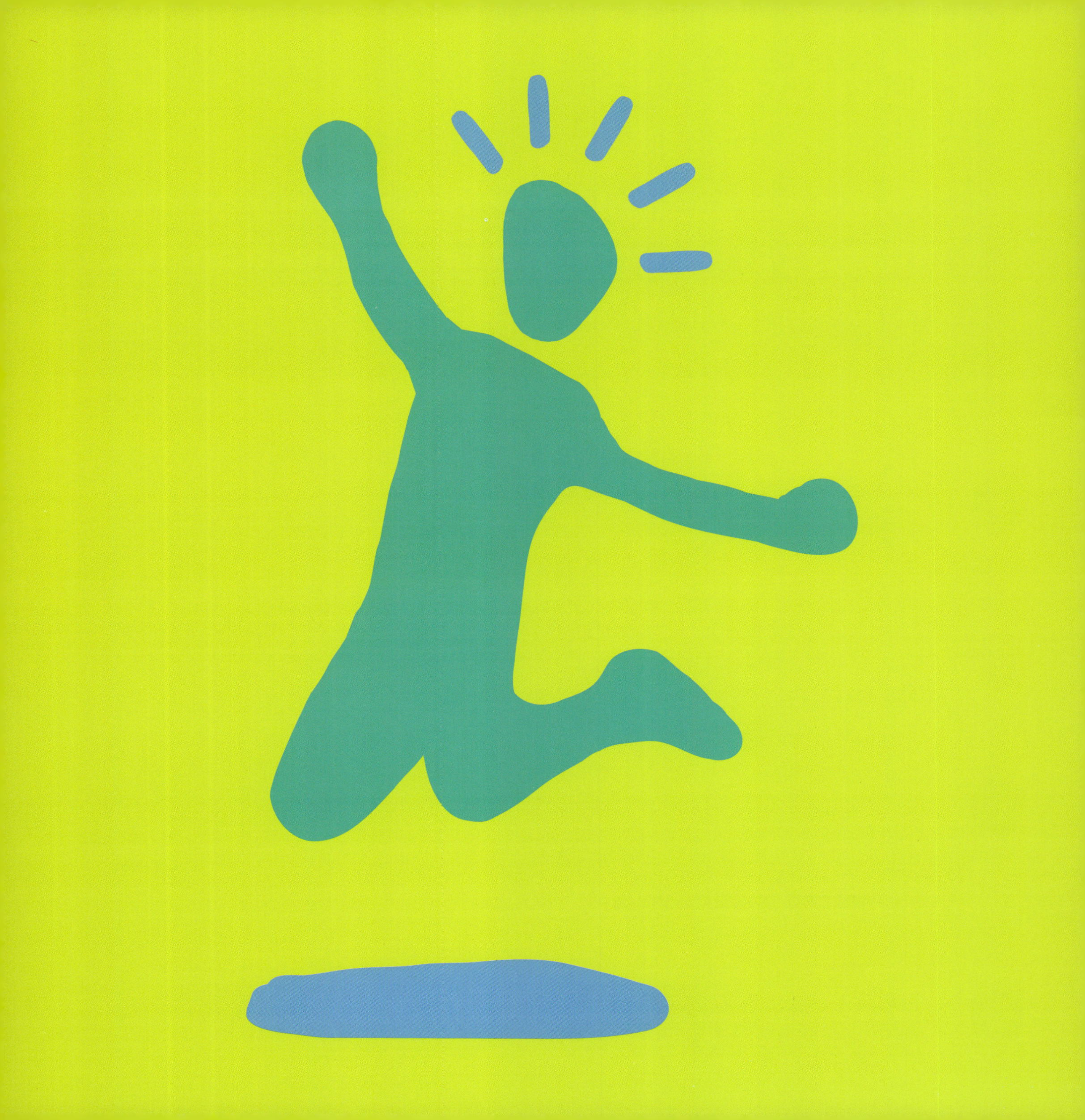

Joy 18

Joy is often seen as the goal itself, but it can also be viewed as the reward for an independent goal, a carrot to a life ambition or a work stick.

Joy, a positive pleasurable, often short term experience, can be the reward for a simple effort. Full long term sustainable happiness is the product of a long term commitment to building a more robust comprehensive personal wellbeing.

Joy versus Happiness. How do you feel about a life that gives you continued pleasure, a confident disposition and a social life that keeps giving amongst caring friends versus a life of quick self-indulgent experiences that offer elastoplast solutions?

The benefits of joy and **positive warm experiences** in your life are often obvious and can become the ambition. However, we probably need a long term strategy to manage and maintain these experiences in preference to a short burst.

"The joy of life comes from our encounters with new experiences, and hence there is no greater joy than to have an endlessly changing horizon, for each day to have a new and different sun."
Christopher McCandless

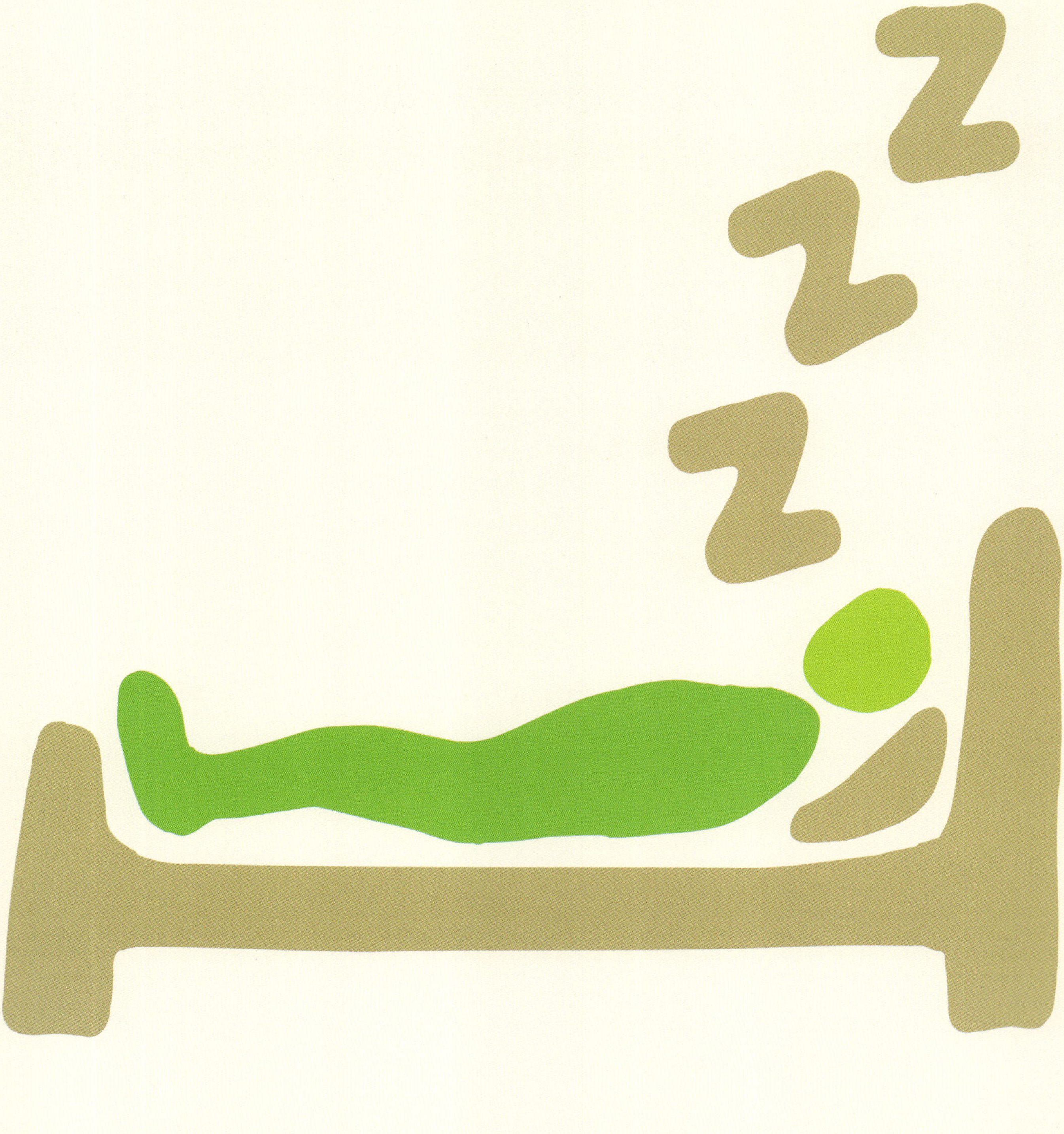
ZZZ

Sleep 19

A full night's sleep prevents ill health, helps reduce stress, improves your mood, allows you to think clearly, improves your sociability and more...

People are now understanding that a full night's sleep is **as important as the other fundamentals such as a good diet and exercise**. The shorter your sleep, the shorter your life span. Sleep is the time your body and mind do essential repairs and maintenance. Human beings are the only species that will deliberately deprive themselves of sleep without legitimate gain. The physical and mental impairments caused by one night of bad sleep dwarf those caused by an equivalent absence of food or exercise.

If you have a bad night's sleep, you could ask someone close to you how it has affected your mood. Ask them whether you were different in any way. Perhaps you were less patient or more irritable?

There are several stages to sleep and science is revealing some core patterns and essential stages throughout the night. It is important to go through all the stages of sleep to feel the full benefit. No short cuts.

"Sleep is the single most effective thing we can do to reset our brain and body health each day - Mother Nature's best effort yet at contra-death."
Matthew Walker

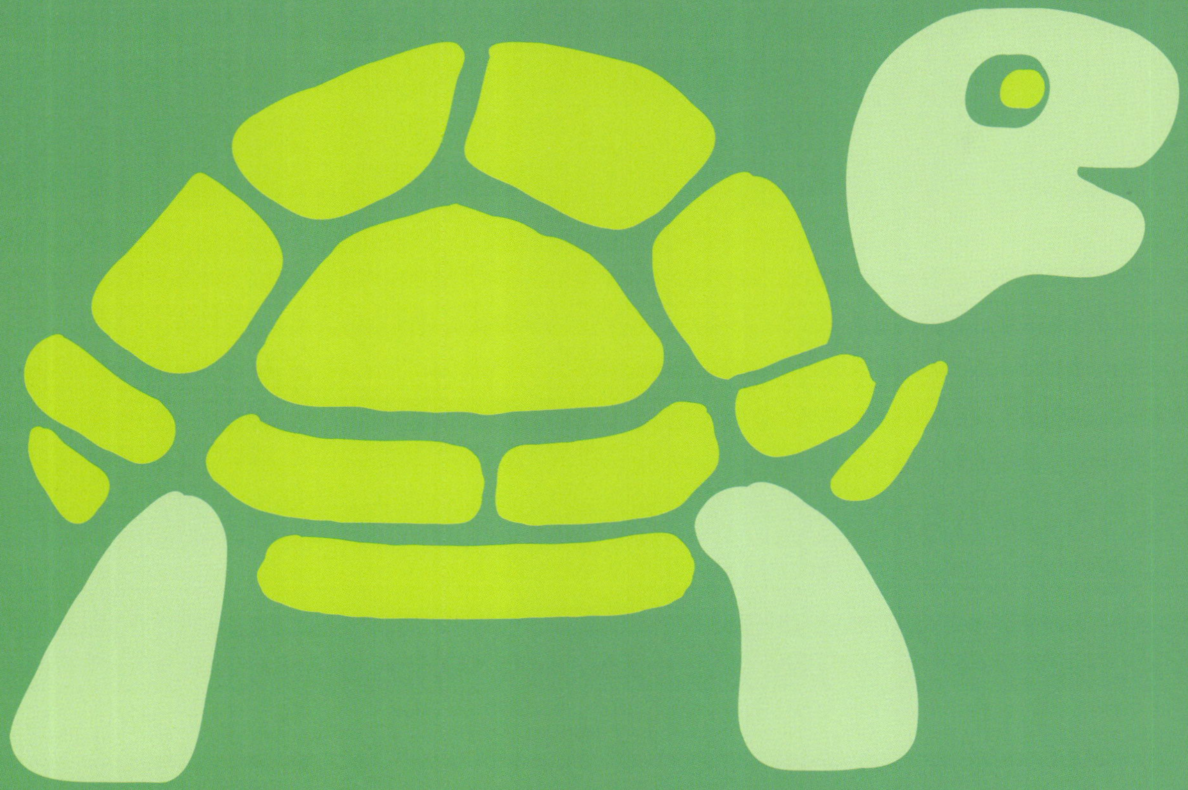

Patience 20

Finding your sense of slow, your patient time amongst the hustle and bustle reveals new unexpected feelings and experiences.

Finding a sense of patience can start by learning not to watch the clock, by setting realistic deadlines for yourself or perhaps finding a new pleasure in carrying out old tasks more thoroughly.

Carry out a task such as making a meal, but give yourself twice the time you normally do, and see how you feel doing this. Setting morning alarm calls for work, though important, can provide a distracting and often negative focus. Try exercises, like early nights, that create bedtime habits that avoid alarm clocks in the morning. Try techniques like counting slowly before giving up on a dull task, or before speaking if you have a tendency to blurt.

By **taking your time to do things at a slower pace** and savouring the experience more fully, personal qualities emerge through the way you are doing what you are doing and what you are feeling.

"Time you enjoy wasting, was not wasted." John Lennon

"Time sometimes flies like a bird, sometimes crawls like a snail; but a man is happiest when he does not even notice whether it passes swiftly or slowly." Ivan Turgenev

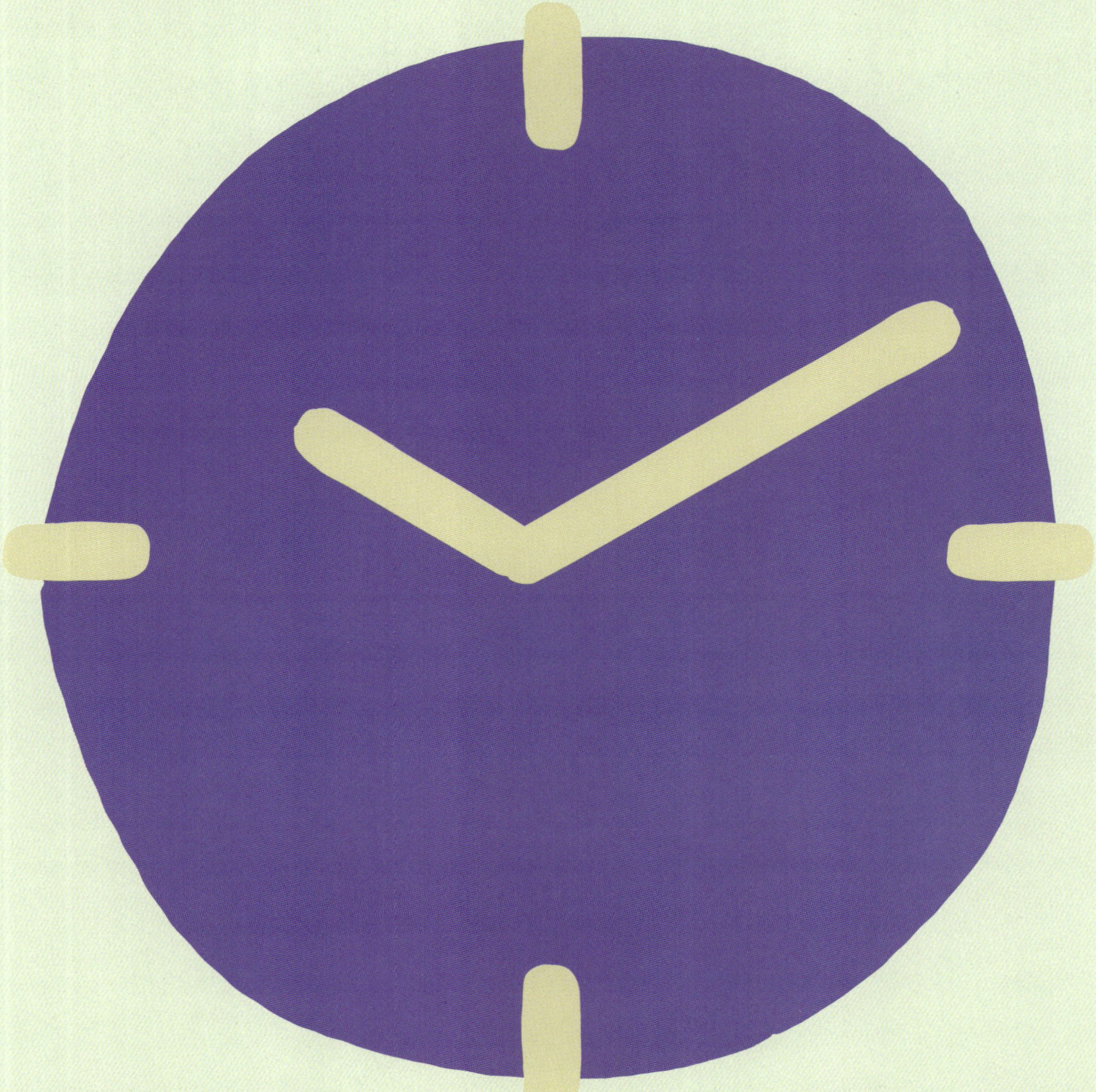

Now 21

The simple action of fully focussing on the immediacy of what you are doing pushes all other thoughts to the edges of your mind.

Being present and embracing mindfulness are becoming more popular forms of finding a state of mind that helps free you from negativity, anxieties and spiralling repetitive thoughts. A simple technique of looking at what you are doing right now, **concentrating on the detail** of a wild flower perhaps, should stop unwanted 'internal dialogue' and give you a necessary break.

Exercise: Stop what you are doing, take a quiet moment to focus on the immediacy of where you are, look at the view, the flower, smell the air, appreciate the detail of this moment and enjoy realising all your worries float to the edges in that moment.

This state of being present and in the moment allows you a breathing space from the day-to-day worries and anxieties that can overwhelm you in a modern hustle and bustle lifestyle.

"Your entire life only happens in this moment. The present moment is life itself. Yet, people live as if the opposite were true and treat the present moment as a stepping stone to the next moment - a means to an end."
Eckhart Tolle

"Living in the now, centreing, being mindful or finding quiet and patience all need practice. Once learnt these techniques can give you a happier life."

“The best feeling in the whole world is the moment you find that inner calm inside yourself and you are truly happy with you.”

3 Summary

Our rest and recreation time is the most valued time we have, as it gives us space to stretch time and make things seem to last a bit longer.

Learning and using new techniques and ways of using our time is a wonderful investment.

Life is short, so every moment we can savour is valuable, stretching this time out, furthering our experiences and enhancing the beauty and detail of all of our lives is amazing.

It is worth taking a little time and investing into new ways of using this, the most precious of all things... time.

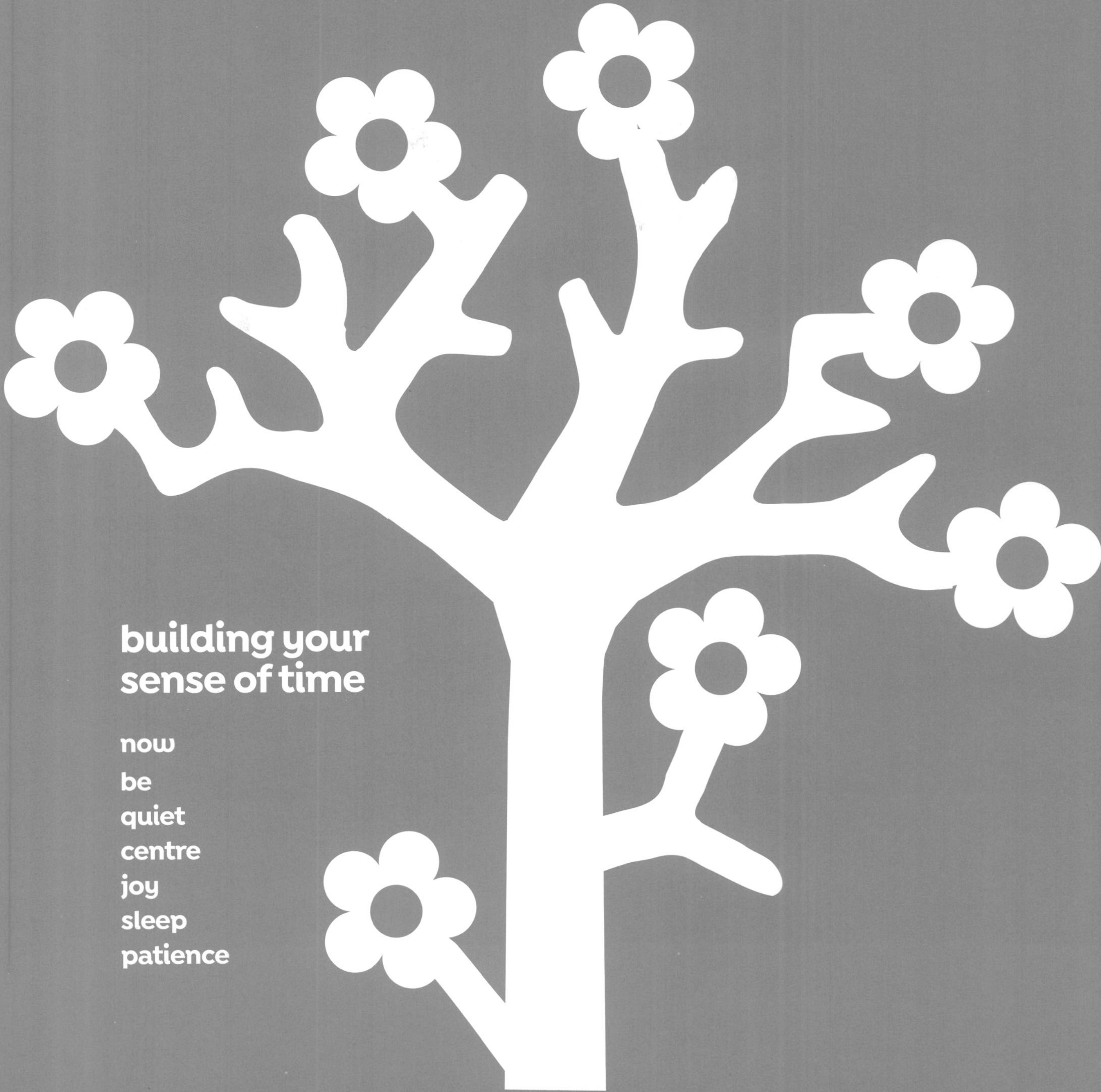

building your sense of time

now
be
quiet
centre
joy
sleep
patience

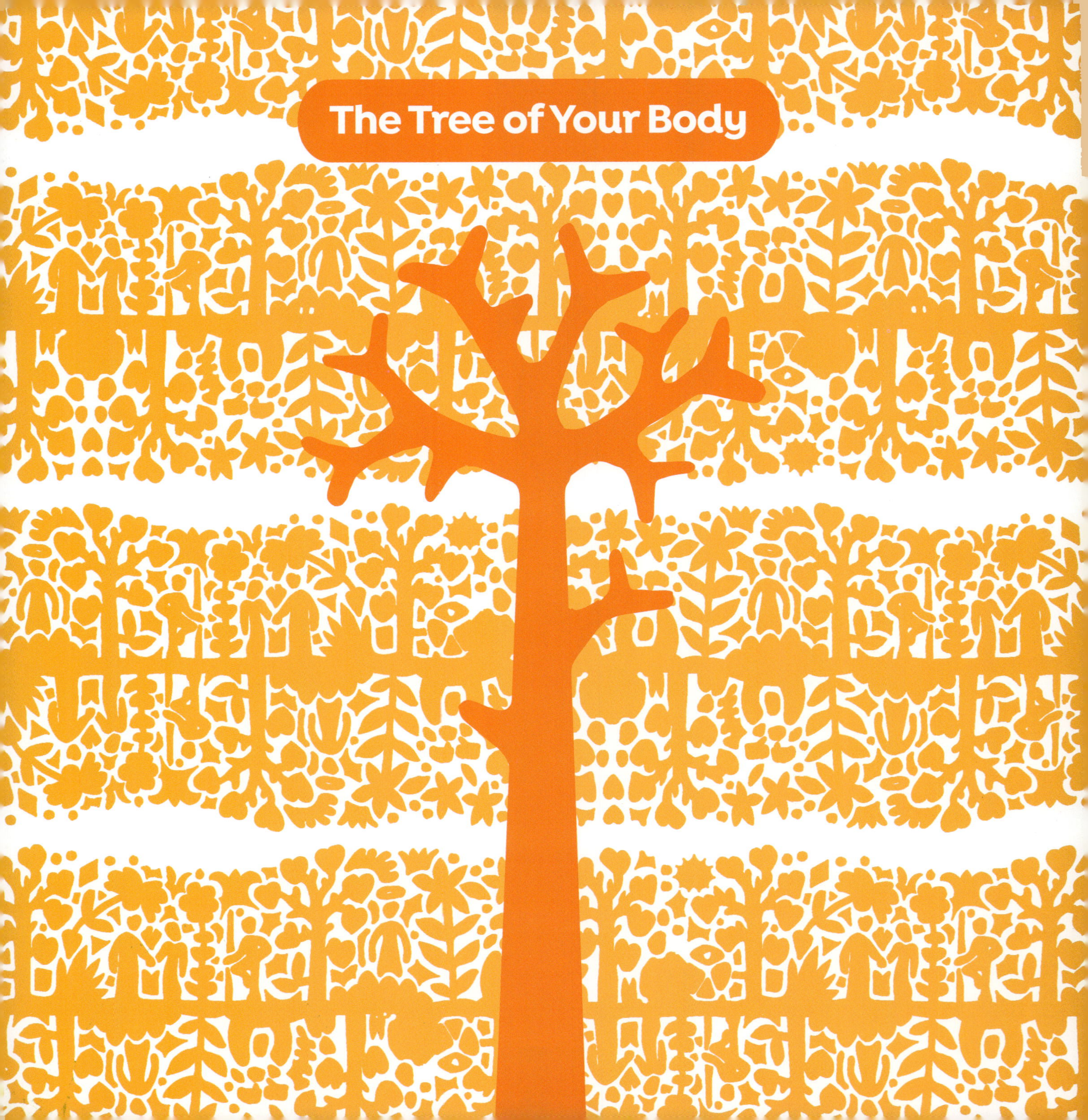
The Tree of Your Body

4

move

drive

needs

balance

building your physical you.

eat

drink

energy

4 Your Body

The Tree of your body, the fourth tree in the Magic Forest of wellbeing is all about understanding and balancing your body.

These words are about building your best physical you, through your physical needs, understanding exercise, movement, motivation, your energy levels, and vitality.

If you work through these key areas and educate yourself carefully on nutrition and hydration then ultimately you can start finding your own ways of achieving a solid healthy physical you and keep it in balance.

The following questions, quotes and insights are a brief summary of the absolute basics required to help you start looking after your body and understanding your body's needs.

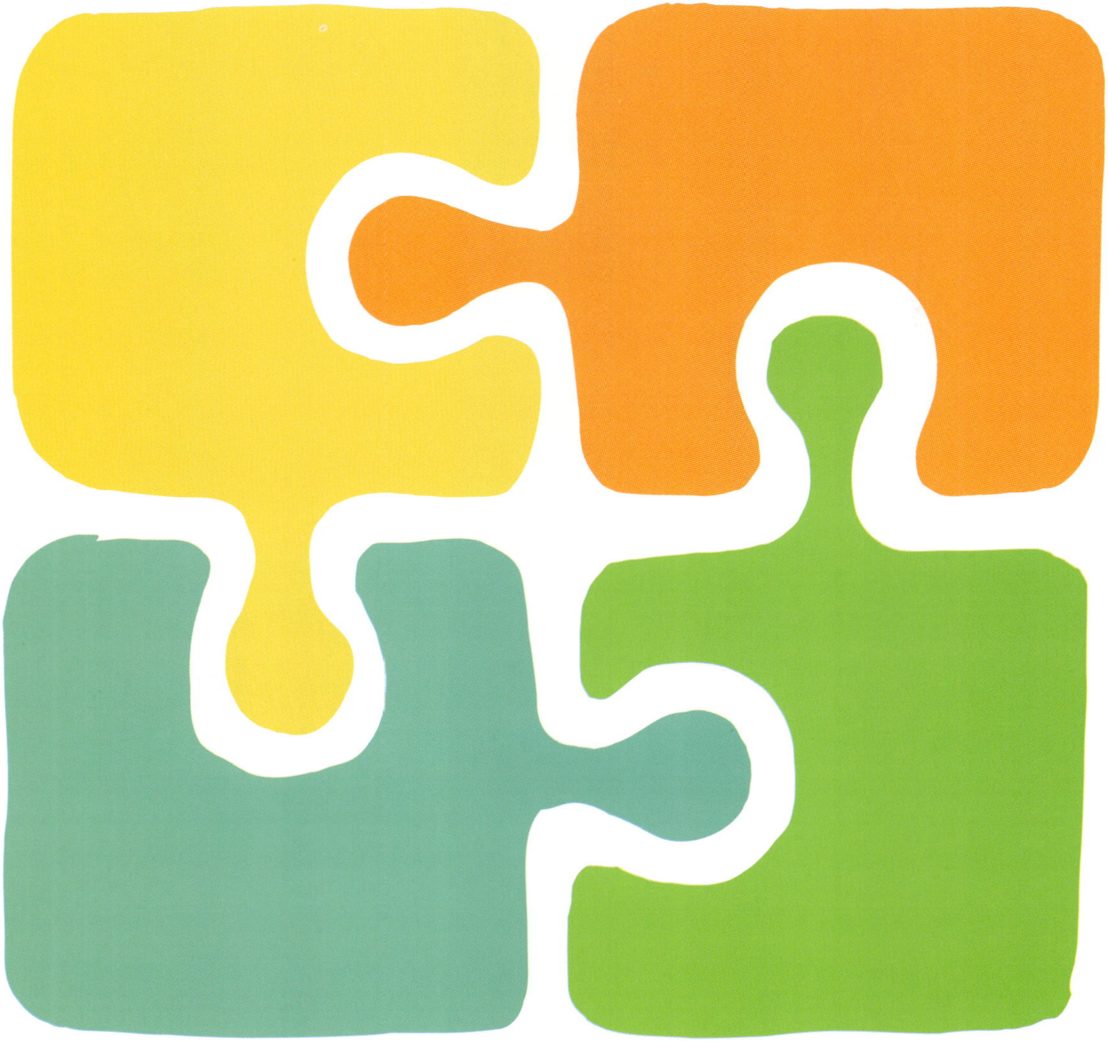

Needs 22

Whatever shape you are or are in, loving and accepting yourself is a vital part of our personal wellbeing. Our self image needs to be nurtured and respected honestly.

We are all different, physically and physiologically and as such we all need to learn a different set of personal requirements. Some people need hours of training, some love routine, some people prefer extreme forms of exercise, diet and motivation. We can only know what we need by **trying things out**, in combination with professional advice of course! If you accept the power of your body and it's million years of evolution to find what is best for it, try and learn to listen for the signals.

Explore different forms of exercise and nutrition, and if it's not your cup of tea, ask yourself why you don't like something. Which foods and exercise really makes your body sing or helps you recover quickly?

The body is an amazing organism and nothing else comes close in terms of just how clever the human mechanisms are that keep it in balance and feedback to the brain to tell you what's going on. Our cells constantly self repair and tissue grows back, imagine something man made that can do that? Wow!

"Pain is your body's way of telling you something is on the edge."

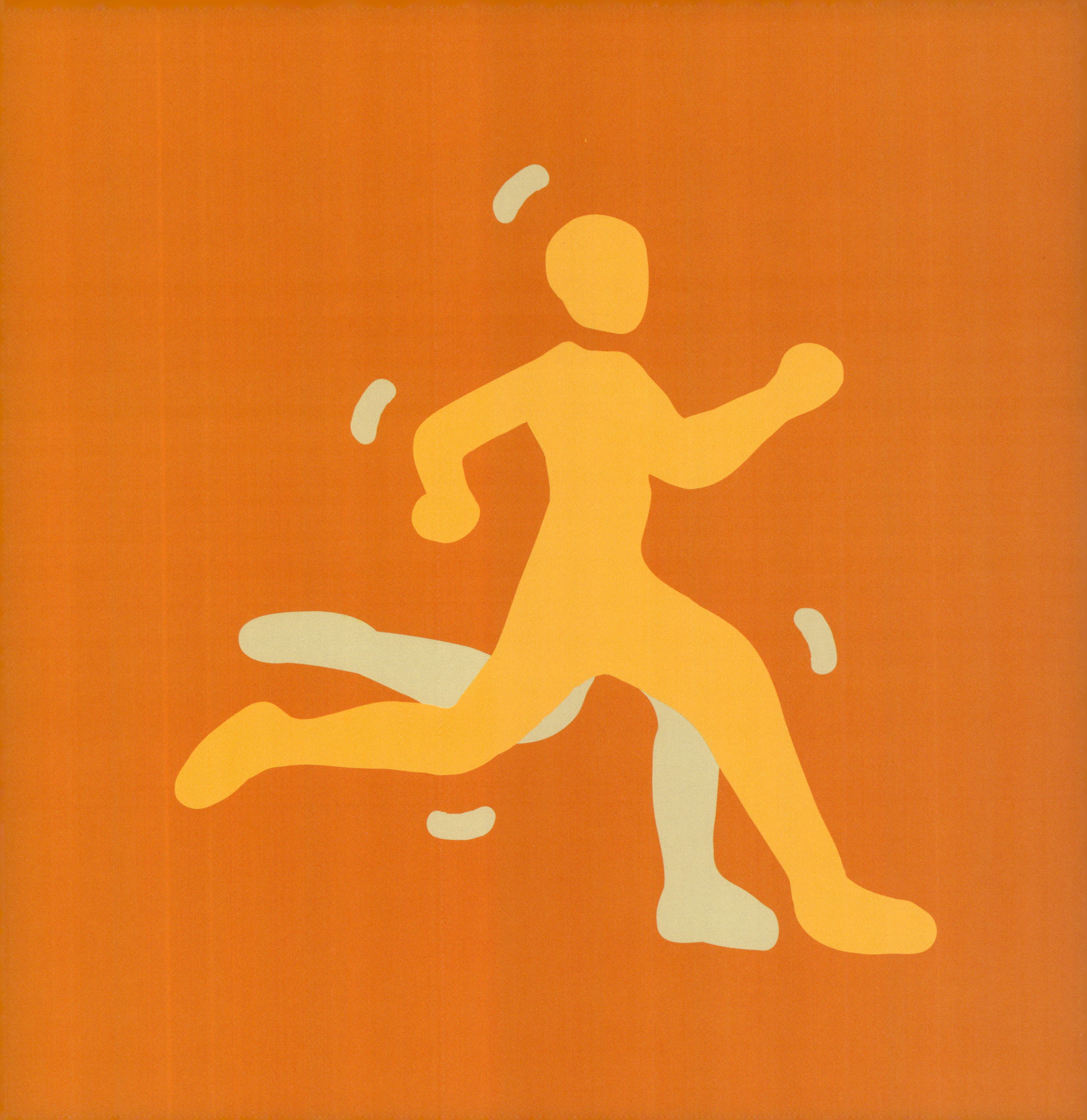

Move 23

Exercise is essential for life. It comes in many forms. A fundamental part of a balanced wellbeing, it may require will power but it definitely must be enjoyed. Go for it!

Find activity you enjoy and do it. Find additional activities you also enjoy and **mix it up**. Make sure it is easy to get up and out and do them. There are a thousand reasons not to exercise and often only one to do it. Look at the basics of the most **valid exercises that raise your heart rate**. Learn about the different types of exercises that build personal strength, stamina or speed. Make the **micro exercises** that are part of your everyday life all add up. These mini workouts like brushing a floor or digging a garden all add precious minutes to your daily routine requirement.

Try leaving your exercise kit all ready by the back door, so that by the time you start finding excuses you are already out there and doing something.

Be honest with your exercise, set goals, build slowly, learn limits and ideally keep a record so you can't kid yourself. Regular is important. A little and often is better than binge.

"Movement is medicine" Anon.

* Disclaimer: These notes are the authors opinion only.
Please consult a Doctor before undertaking any dietary changes or exercise you may be unused to.

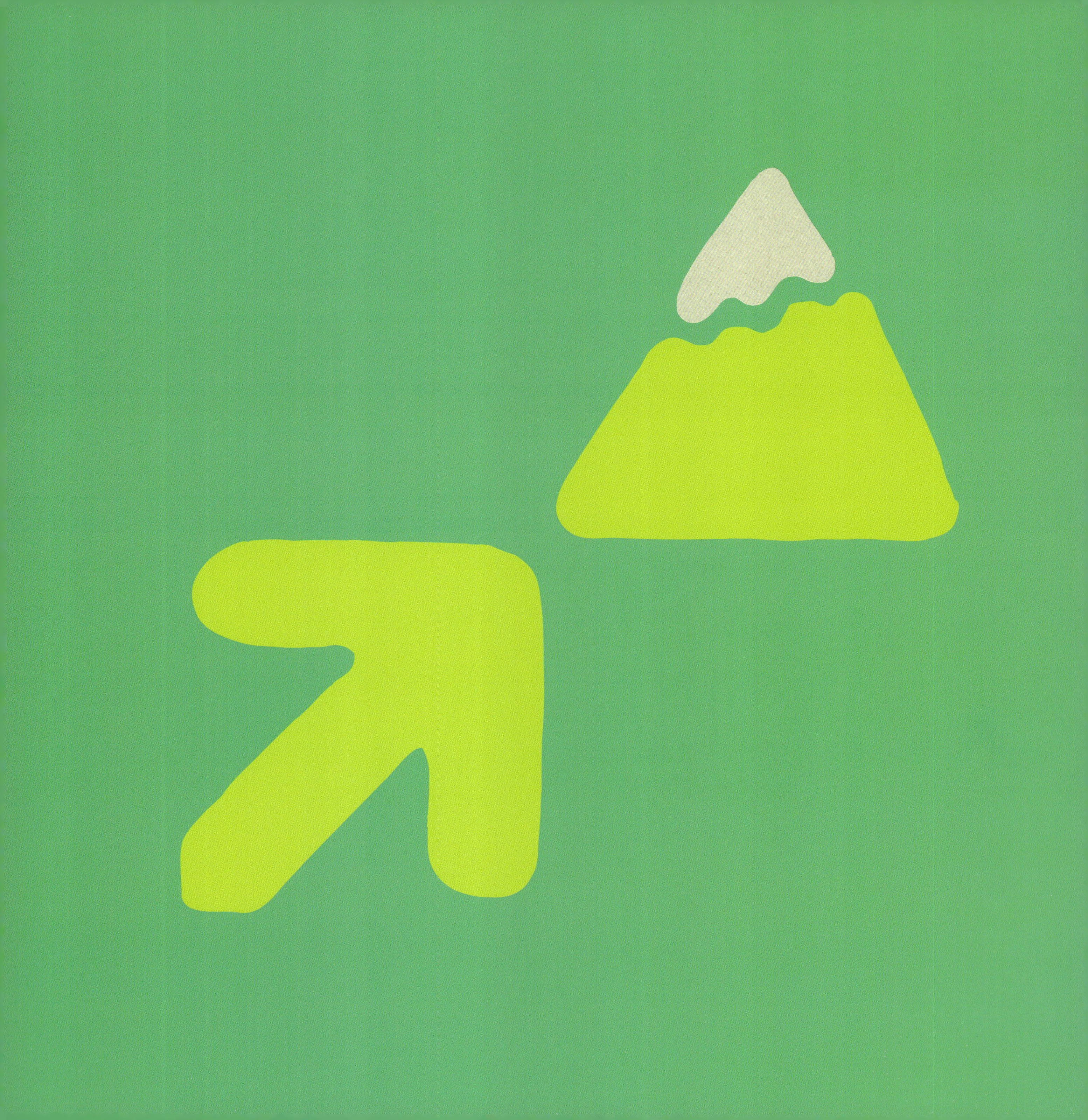

Drive

Finding the motivation to maintain a well-balanced healthy body, our physical self, is key and the answer comes from a great many personal places.

Micro motivations to exercise, micro motivations to manage a good diet, to control calorie intake all need to be kept in check. Keeping everything in check needs a good reason, a motivational thought that drives you. These thoughts are the very personal reasons that keep you going through the tough times. The act of keeping them to yourself can also be quite motivating.

Exercise: Breaking down the steps of a goal is key. Try visualising succeeding at each step and keep the target realistically achievable for each step.

Finding all the things that motivate you to do something is hard, so make sure you find the honest reasons, the **positive motivations** and you will **increase the chances of success** in your endeavour and be able to play a long game. Don't forget to pace yourself and manage each step with a reward, however small, to maintain the motivation.

"Focusing on a long-term goal can be disheartening when you're so far away from it, so it's vital to have ongoing targets on a daily, weekly and monthly basis." Sir Chris Hoy

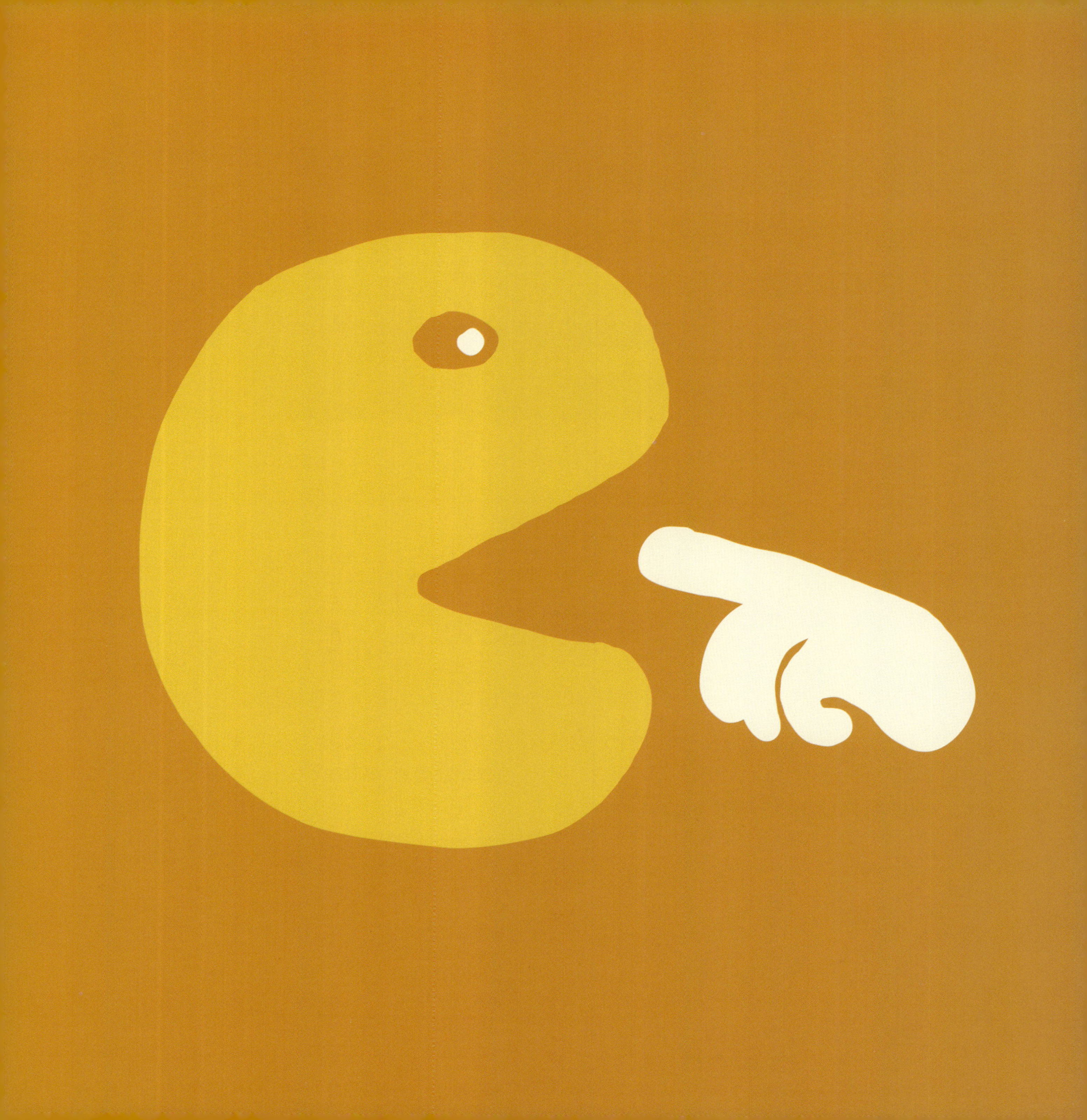

Eat 25

Good food is basically well-balanced nutrition. It is one of the key cornerstones of a strong overall wellbeing. Food is fun.

Diet and the need for good food seems unnecessarily complicated by everything you read in the media. We all have a different opinion. We all have as many different needs as we have lifestyles, but it can be as simple as: Eat a **balanced** diet that comprises essential **vitamins** and a **spread of food types.** Eat as much **unprocessed** food as possible. Stick to foodstuffs that you know where they came from and are as close to the earth as possible. Minimise the obvious high calorie treats and don't deny yourself completely.

Keeping an honest food diary is a great thing to do. You can see where you are lacking in food stuffs and compare it to your energy, exercise or general health wellbeing levels.

Your immune system is affected to a large degree by your diet and is important for your physical wellbeing. A healthy diet, whether it's for calories or nutrition, helps build and maintain this system, and is always best when it is both sustainable and enjoyable.

"Healthy eating is a way of life, so it's important to establish routines that are simple, realistically, and ultimately livable." Horace

* Disclaimer: These notes are the authors opinion only.
Please consult a Doctor before undertaking any dietary changes or exercise you may be unused to.

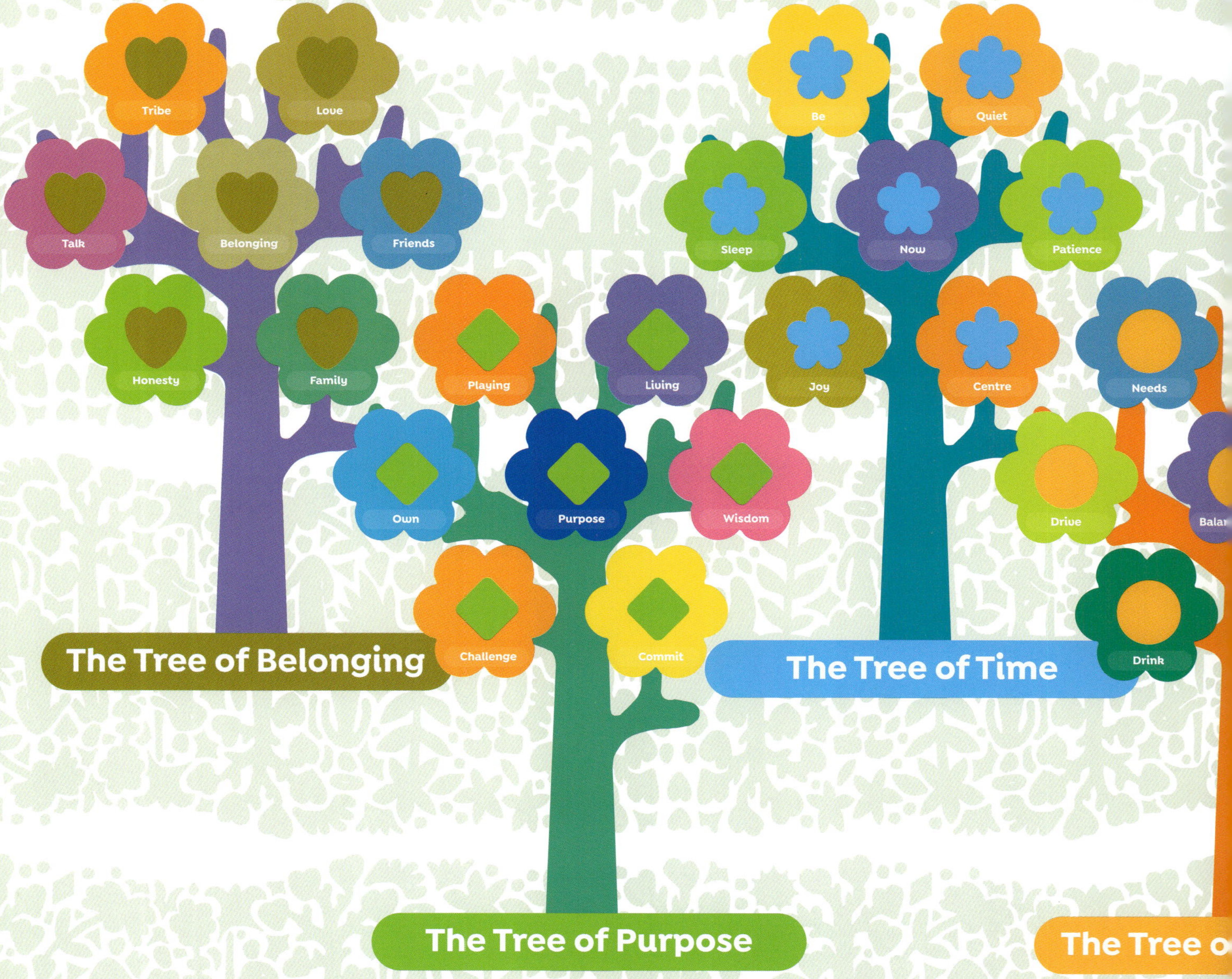
Tribe
Love
Talk
Belonging
Friends
Honesty
Family
The Tree of Belonging
Playing
Living
Own
Purpose
Wisdom
Challenge
Commit
The Tree of Purpose
Be
Quiet
Sleep
Now
Patience
Joy
Centre
The Tree of Time
Needs
Drive
Drink

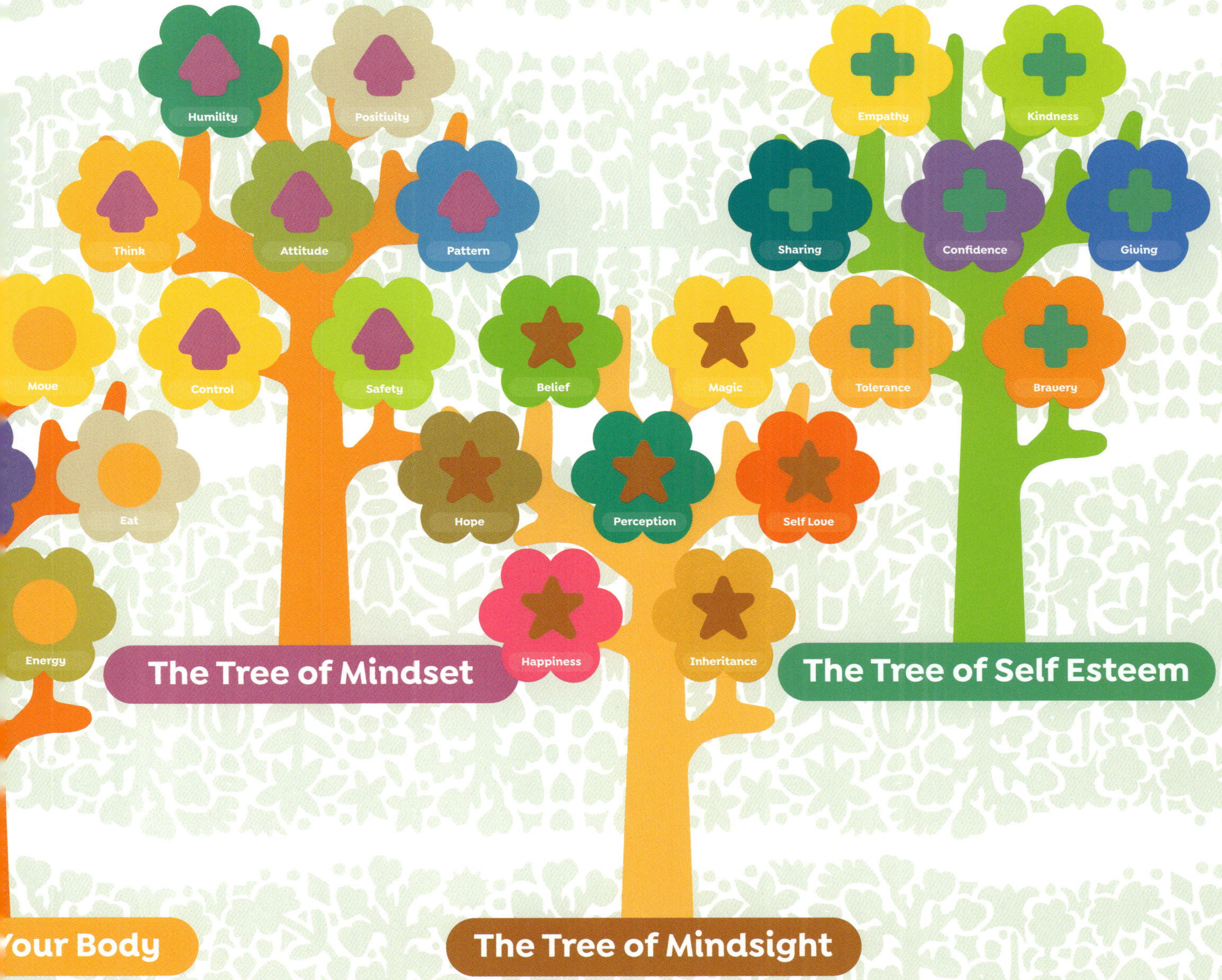

as if by magic... a forest appears.

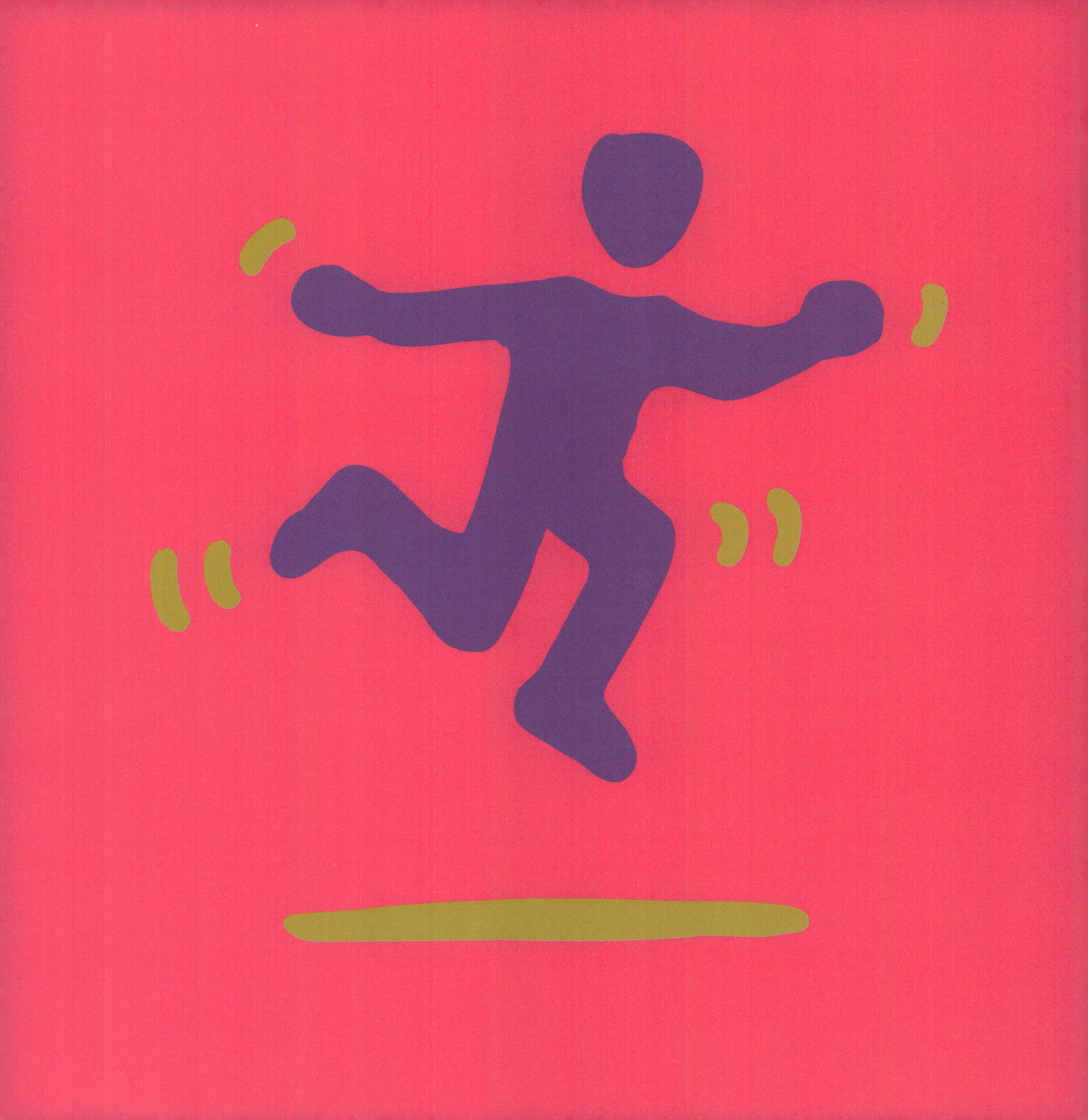

Energy

26

It is a strange quirk of nature that the more exercise you do the more energy you have to do other things. I call it the exercise-energy paradox, you might call it bonkers.

Feeling vital and having the 'get up and go' energy can be trained, and it isn't necessarily lost with age. Diet, exercise and overall care for your body and mind, is precisely the aim of this small book of wellbeing and one of the major benefits of looking after your exercise and diet is the amount of energy you have for other things.

Try a simple exercise of a great diet and some more than usual exercise for a week or two then, after recovery, measure your work output and ask yourself how vigorous you were at work?

Having the passion or **energy for everything that life brings** to you is the greatest feeling. However, as with so many things in life, there are no quick fixes or real shortcuts and this vitality is the great reward for all your investment in all the other aspects of your wellbeing especially a balanced diet and regular exercise.

"Be fired with passion or be fired with passion" My wonderful dad

"Get up and Go, before it's got up and gone!" Anon

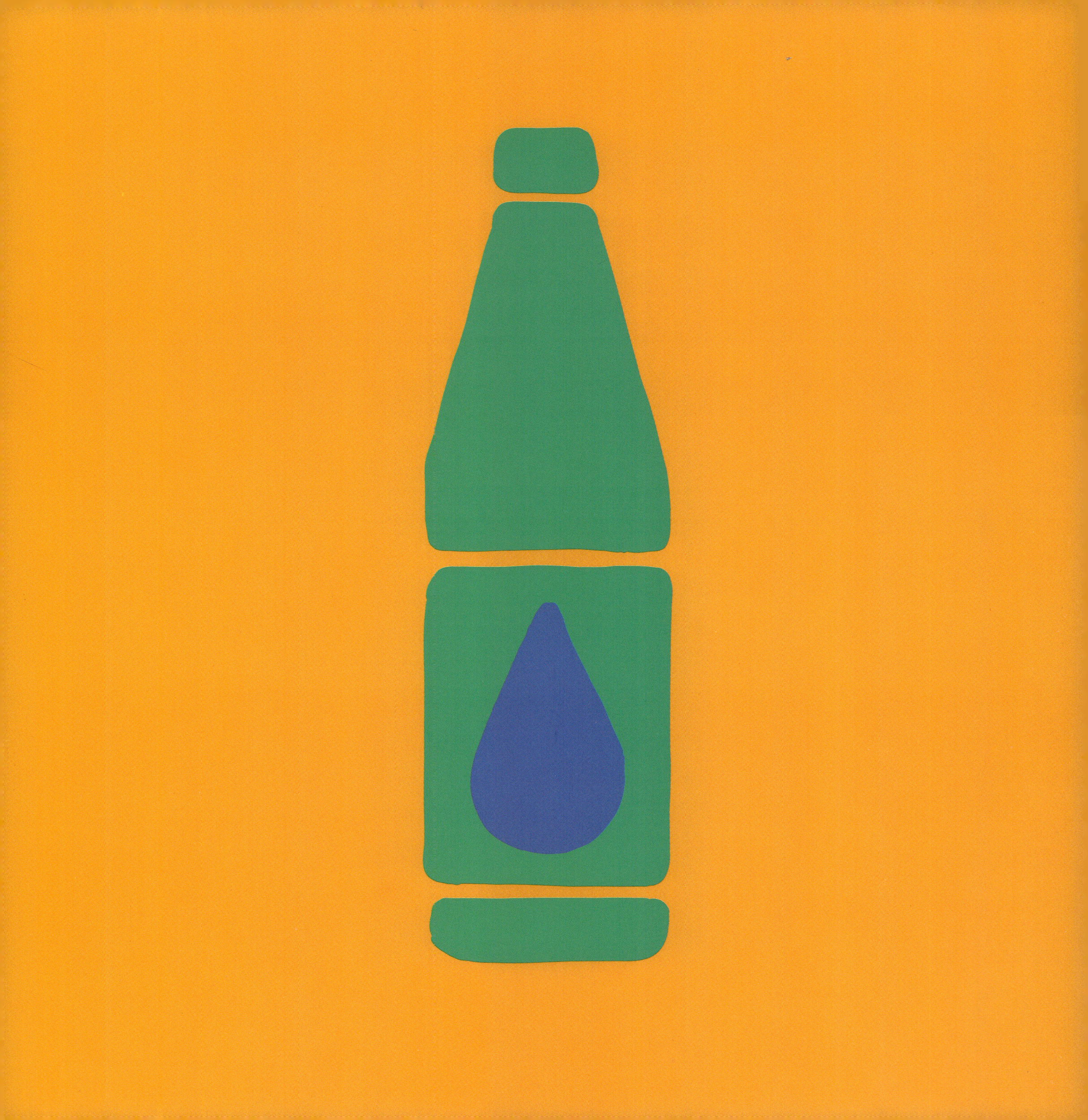

Drink

27

Drinking correctly is a cornerstone of good health. Good hydration means you balance the fluids you lose with those you take in. Many wonderful, flawed people get this wrong. Hic.

If you are thirsty, you are probably already dehydrated. Major causes of dehydration include alcohol consumption as well as not drinking enough **water throughout the day**. Sugary drinks, tea and coffee may just dehydrate you.

Exercise: Try using a water bottle and keeping it close at hand. Flavoured water can provide variety and an incentive.

Drinking enough water each day is crucial for many reasons: to regulate body temperature, keep joints lubricated, prevent infections, deliver nutrients to cells, and keep organs functioning properly. Being well-hydrated also improves sleep quality, cognition, and mood.

"Drink! for you know not whence you came nor why: drink! for you know not why you go, nor where." Omar Khayyam

"It takes only one drink to get me drunk. The trouble is, I can't remember if it's the thirteenth or the fourteenth." George Burns

* Disclaimer: These notes are the authors opinion only.
Please consult a Doctor before undertaking any dietary changes or exercise you may be unused to.

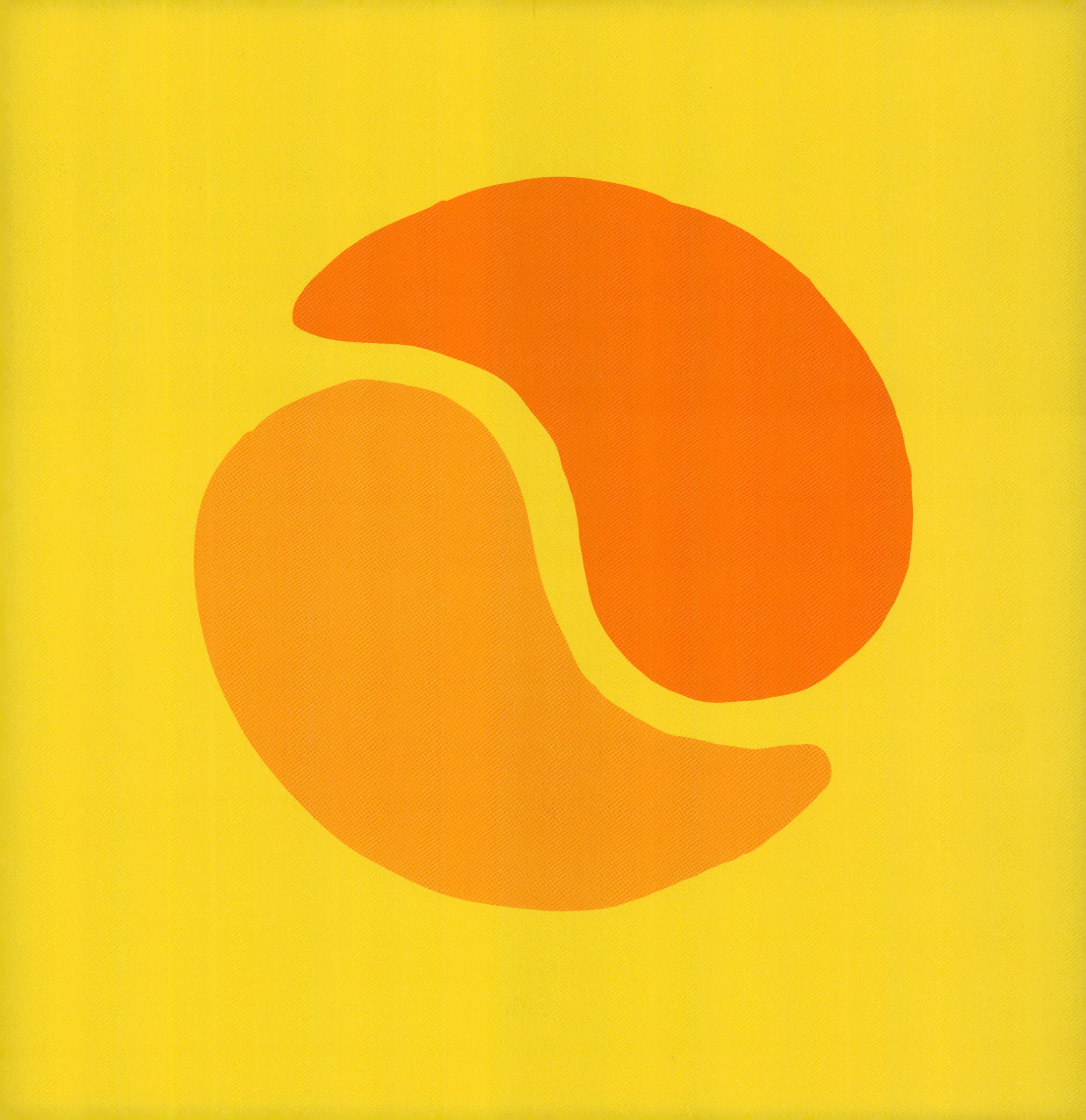

Balance 28

The human being repairs itself! Your body, if looked after with food and water properly, can repair and rebuild cells to new overnight. This alone should give cause for awe.

Reaching a balanced physical wellbeing is as amazing as it is rare. For most of our young lives this is automatic, inbuilt and happens without us knowing or even feeling it. Key to getting older is understanding both sides of your personal input-output equation. Balancing exercise, lifestyle, healthy food and managing your immune system with your correct ratio healthy foodstuff including essential vitamins to exercise output.

Listening to your body is key. Learn the language of how it works. For example, pain is your body's way of saying something is wrong. Ask yourself what are nature's other forms of communication between your brain and your body.

The most sophisticated organism on this planet is driven by a brain that has more than 100 trillion connections, so the least we can do is care a little about food input and exercise output!

"Learn to love and accept your body for all its wonder, shape and size, it is yours and without a shadow of a doubt it's the only one you're going to get." Anon.

“Your body will tell you everything. The important thing is to learn to listen.”

“It doesn’t matter what shape you are or are in, it’s the fact you are doing something about improving your life that really matters – and you should always feel good that you are.”

4 Summary

Our preoccupation with our bodies is as old as history itself, but these notes aren't about all that. These pages are a celebration of the wonders of everything that makes us physical us.

The frame we all own carries us through life and for the most part doesn't complain when we look after it. Even when we push it through everyday life's thousands of steps and take it on extreme adventures to the furthest flung places, it adapts.

The trouble all starts when we don't realise what an unbelievable miracle of a gift we have all been bestowed. A gift that literally keeps on giving for a lifetime, self repairing and managing to do extraordinary things when we forget to feed it, water it and even occasionally smash it traumatically into pieces, as in this authors' case.

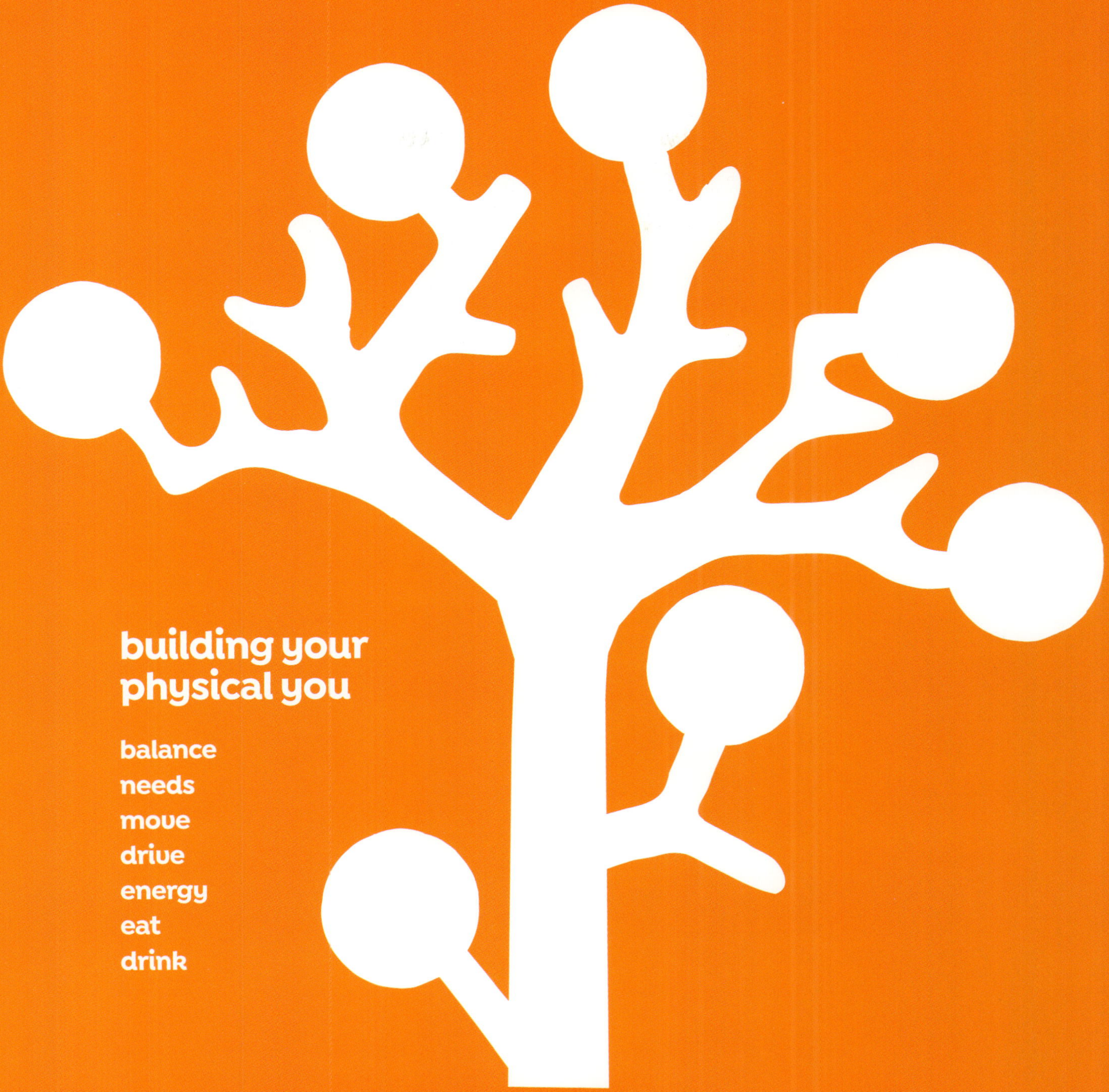

building your physical you

balance
needs
move
drive
energy
eat
drink

The Tree of Mindset

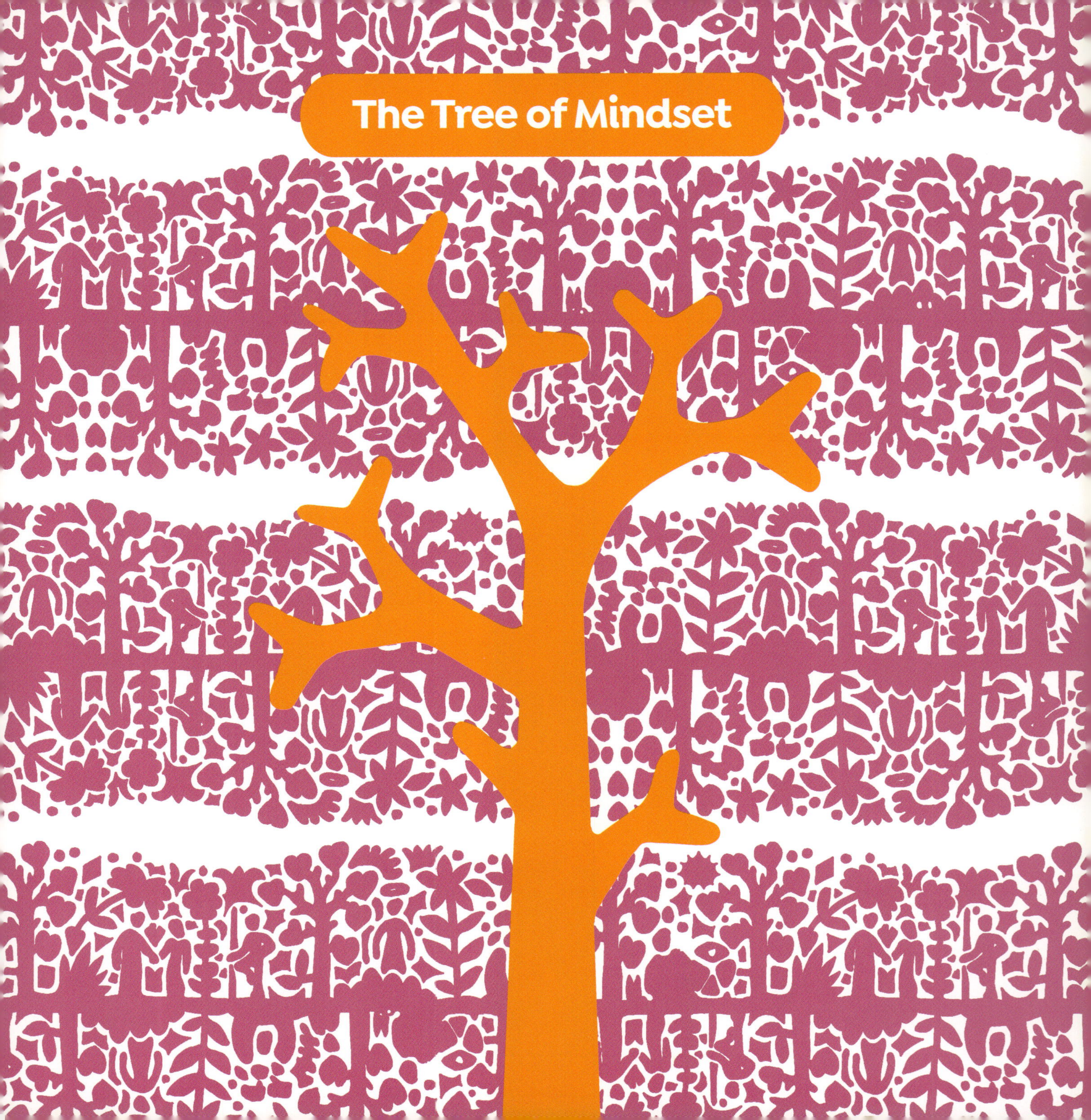

5

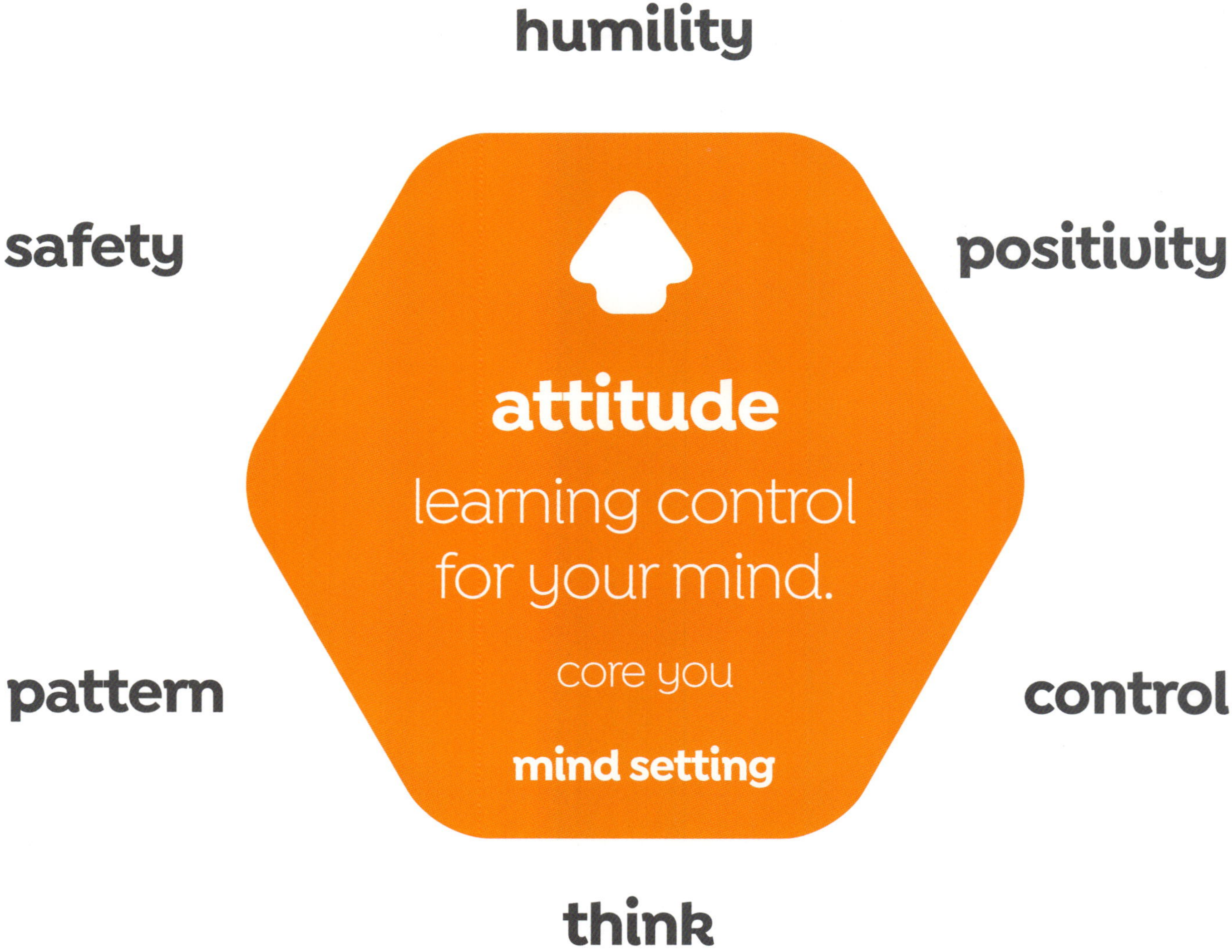
humility
safety
positivity
attitude
learning control
for your mind.
core you
mind setting
pattern
control
think

5 Your Mindset

The Tree of Mindset is the fifth in the Magic Forest and is all about learning control of, and living happily with, your mind.

These words help build your understanding that you are in control of your thoughts and can learn to love them, finding a safe place in your mind to happily spend time with them.

The mindset tree should help you recognise that some thoughts are only thoughts. By anticipating the patterns of your thoughts, finding positivity, developing consideration, humility and a good attitude, you can build a stronger mental wellbeing for yourself.

The following questions, quotes and insights are a summary of essential elements to help you start building your understanding, questioning and learning about your mind and mindset.

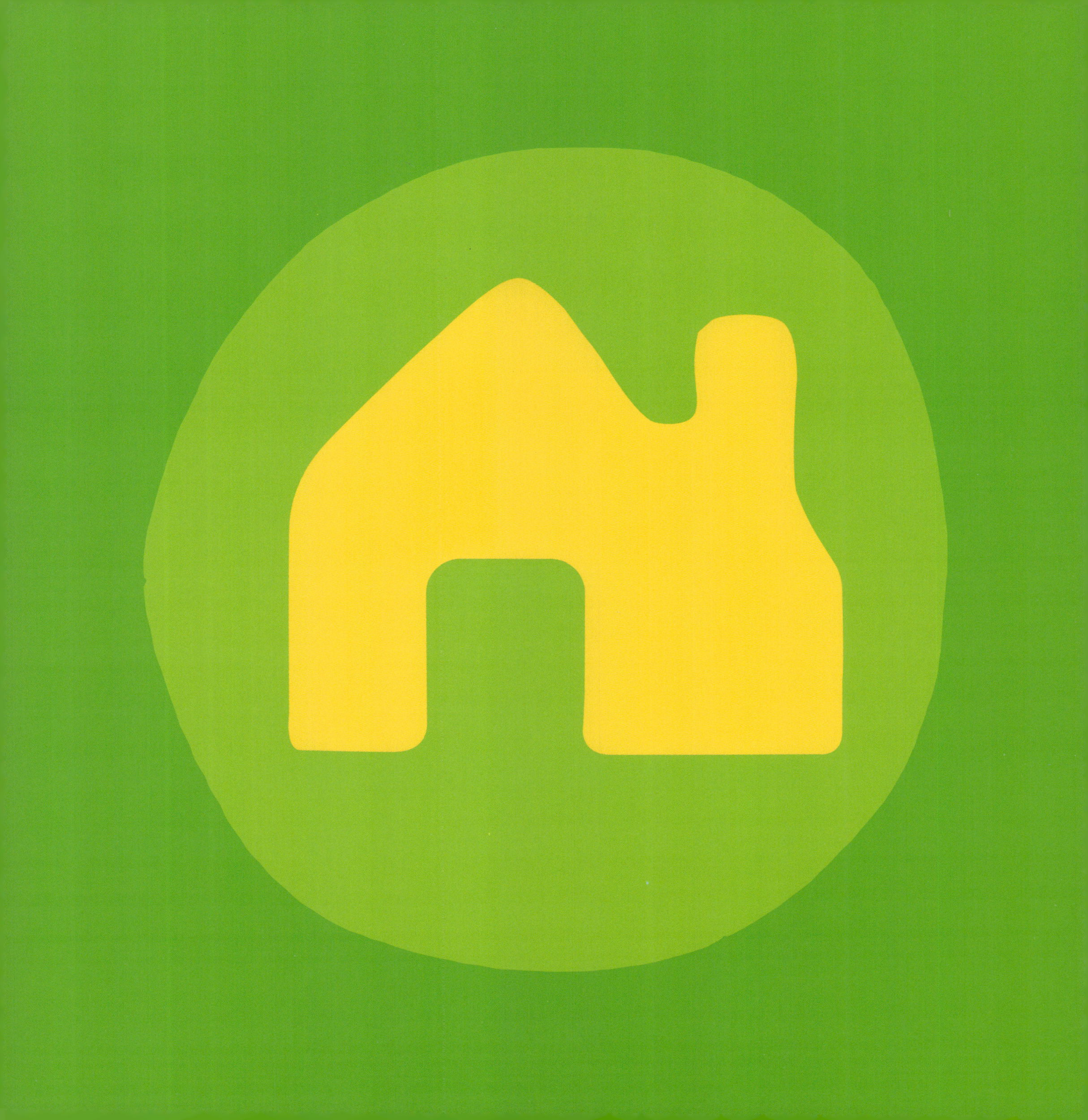

Safety 29

Home is a safe place to live your life from, a reassuring comfortable base to explore the world out there. Making a similar place in your mind is key to finding mental strength.

If the answer to 'how do you feel about yourself these days?' is 'I like me, I'm OK, I'm a decent kind of person and **I can sleep at night** knowing I have done some good out there' then chances are you have a safe comfortable mind up top and you probably aren't reading this. The rest of us have to aspire to be you and find our own sanctuary in the mind, we need to find some things about ourselves we love and respect, to set a flag in the ground and keep coming back to it, however small.

Try asking yourself, 'What makes me feel good about me and makes me feel strong inside?'

This positive self image of yourself can give you a **calm sanctuary in your mind** which comes with a calm external disposition. A smile from within will shine through and the greater this is your own sense of self and the less this is for others the better you will feel.

"The more one does and sees and feels, the more one is able to do, and the more genuine may be one's appreciation of fundamental things like home, and love, and understanding companionship." Amelia Earhart

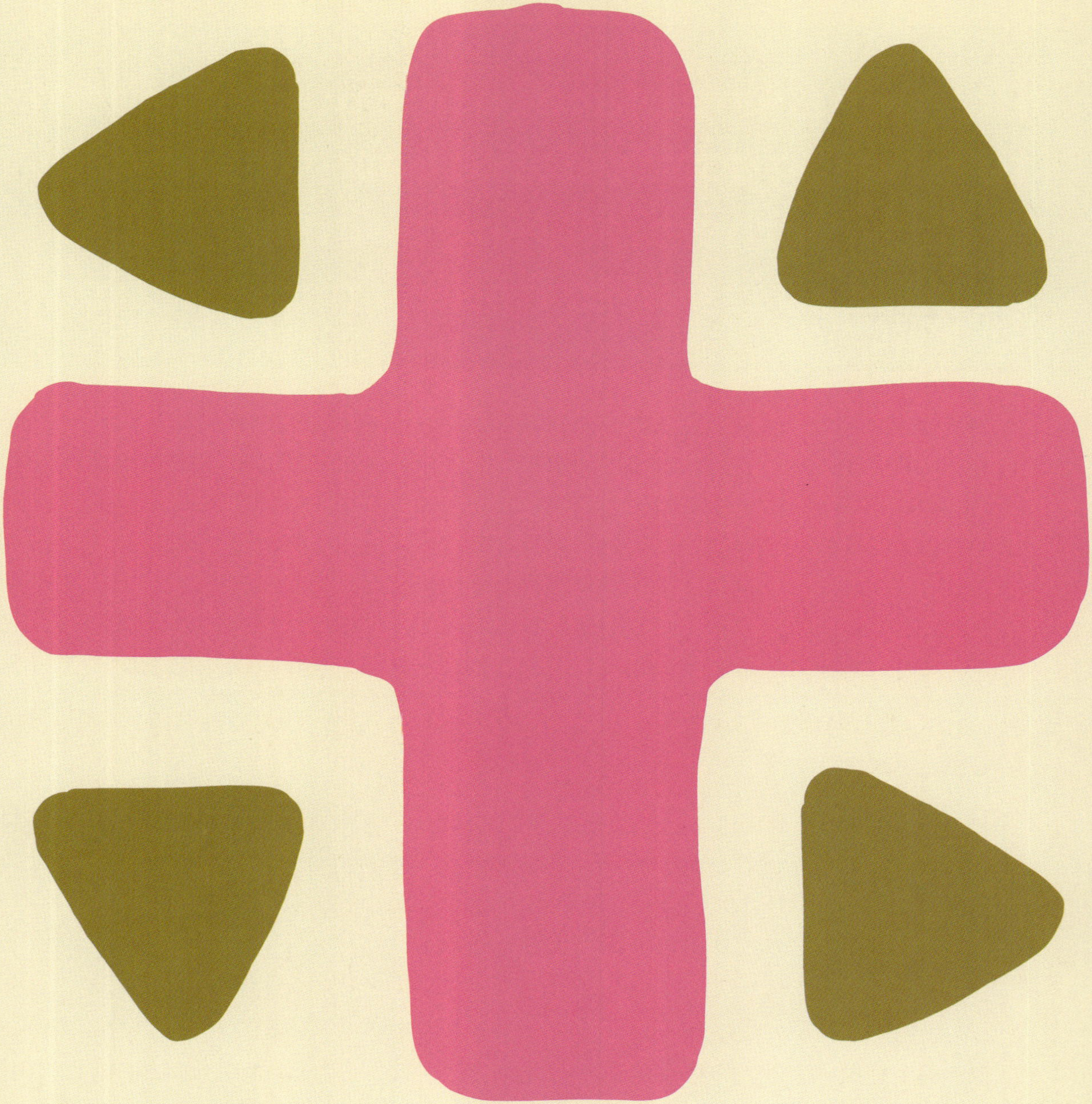

Positivity 30

Positive thoughts come from thoughts that are neutral and you have decided to make them positive - you are in control. You only have to decide how to do this.

Positivity and the whole glass half full thing is often just a **new way of looking at things.** It is as easy to look at your problems as your opportunities and vice versa. Taking this time to make sure they don't happen again or become a recurring theme can be a great investment.

Find a technique that works for you to encourage positive thoughts. (This could be 'cognitive behaviour therapy' - CBT). A simple physical action such as shaking your head when you have an unwanted thought can encourage you to consciously find a more positive one. Eventually you can do it without the action.

Basically, if you look at everything you can and find the positive in it, it often becomes a positive - a self-fulfilling prophecy.

"You are the sum total of everything you've ever seen, heard, eaten, smelled, been told, forgot - it's all there. Everything influences each of us, and because of that I try to make sure that my experiences are positive." Maya Angelou

"The way positive reinforcement is carried out is more important than the amount." B. F. Skinner

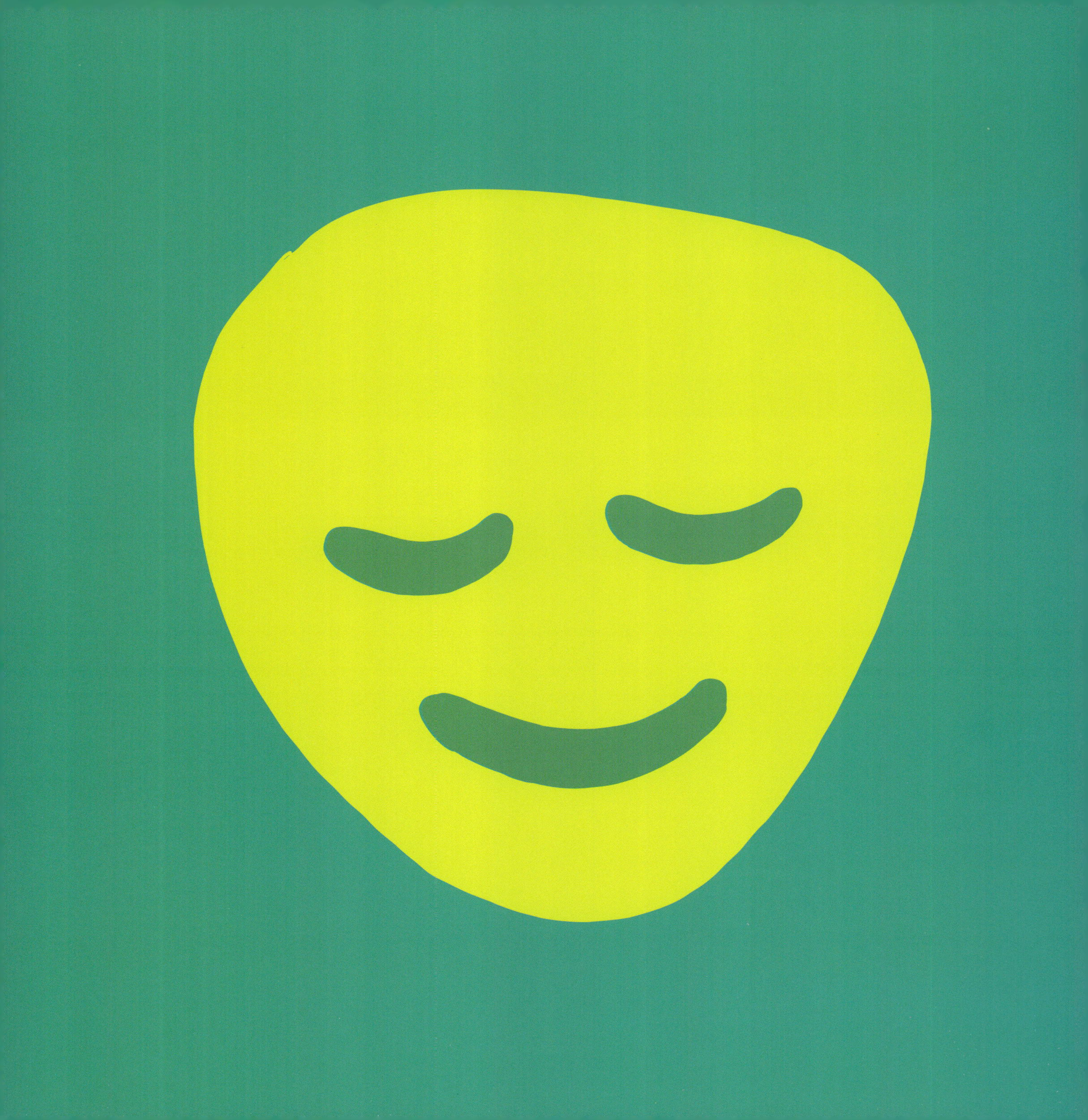

Humility

31

We are all individuals, we all have an opinion so it stands to reason these will probably be different. Humility is this acceptance.

Learning to find humility through accepting other people's opinions, and that they may be as important to them as yours are to you, is the common ground that ensures you will be an altogether more accepting and a subsequently more sociable human being.

Take the time to stand back from a person and perhaps park your initial judgements and opinions and think empathetically about **what that person has been through in their life to make them behave in the way they do?** Often you will find respect and feel humbled, which in turn makes you more endearing as you have taken a moment and started to understand and respect them.

Hubris or runaway over confidence and a strong belief in your own ways is the opposite of humility. The middle ground of humility, of confidence in your own opinions, yet not forcibly pushing them on others is a great way of building a strong group of genuine friends.

"True empathy is rooted in humility and the understanding that there are many people with as much to contribute in life as you." Anand Mahindra

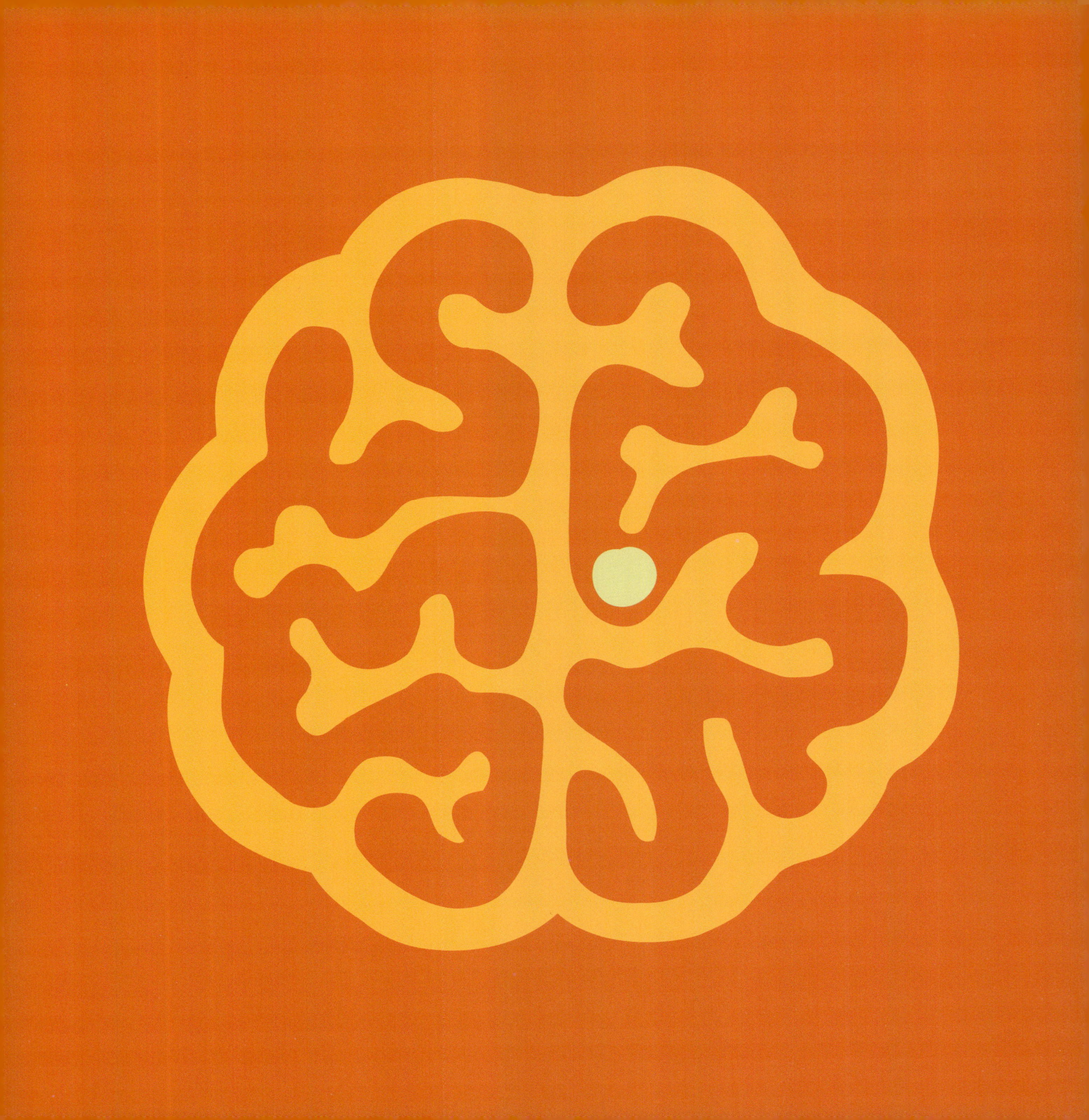

Think 32

Becoming more considered, looking around and taking into consideration other people's thoughts and ideas leads to stronger decisions.

Taking the time to think about your problems and a decision you have to make is an ideal, albeit often elusive, way of tackling life choices. The more time you can manage to take to think through each step, the stronger the eventuality or outcome.

Ask yourself 'Have I considered all aspects of this problem, have I done my best?' If the answer is yes then you will have probably made a good decision, you won't regret in the future and will sleep more easily. You could see the time spent as an investment in your peace of mind in the future. Your mental wellbeing.

If **you are a product of your life decisions**, and you can make these as well as possible, you are making a big contribution to your peace of mind. That you have done your best and made the best decision at that time for you feels great.

"Too often we enjoy the comfort of opinion without the discomfort of thought." John F. Kennedy

"Learning without thought is labour lost; thought without learning is perilous." Confucius

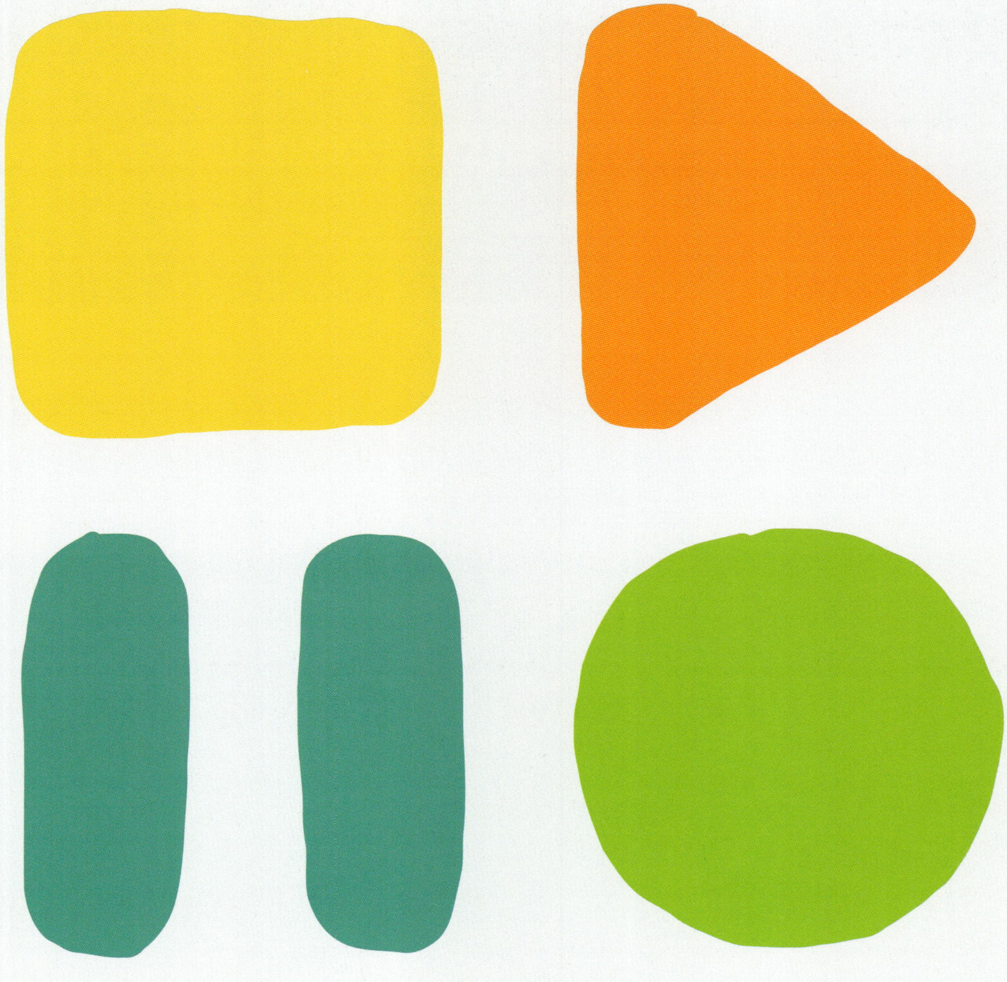

Control 33

You are in control of your own thoughts. You have control over whether you choose to think further about them or not. The challenge is becoming the person you want to be.

Thoughts can occur randomly and spontaneously for everybody. As such, however good or even frightening they may be, they can be recognised as just another perhaps harmless thought. They need to be encouraged or ignored appropriately. The key is to learn to trust your mind's thoughts.

Learn to respect your internal dialogue. By only saying things to yourself you believe and mean, then you can build this internal respect.

Learning to trust your mind won't run out of control and say something you don't really believe is an important lesson to learn. The anxiety that you might give away true inner feelings can be a big fear until you have learnt you are in control. A good solution is to befriend your mind and enjoy the privileges of this inner trust in conversation. When you **know who you are** and have built your inner confidence, then you are much more likely to speak the truth of you and then be seen as your best self.

"I can control my destiny, but not my fate." Paulo Coelho

"You cannot control what happens to you, but you can control your attitude toward what happens to you, and in that, you will be mastering change rather than allowing it to master you." Brian Tracy

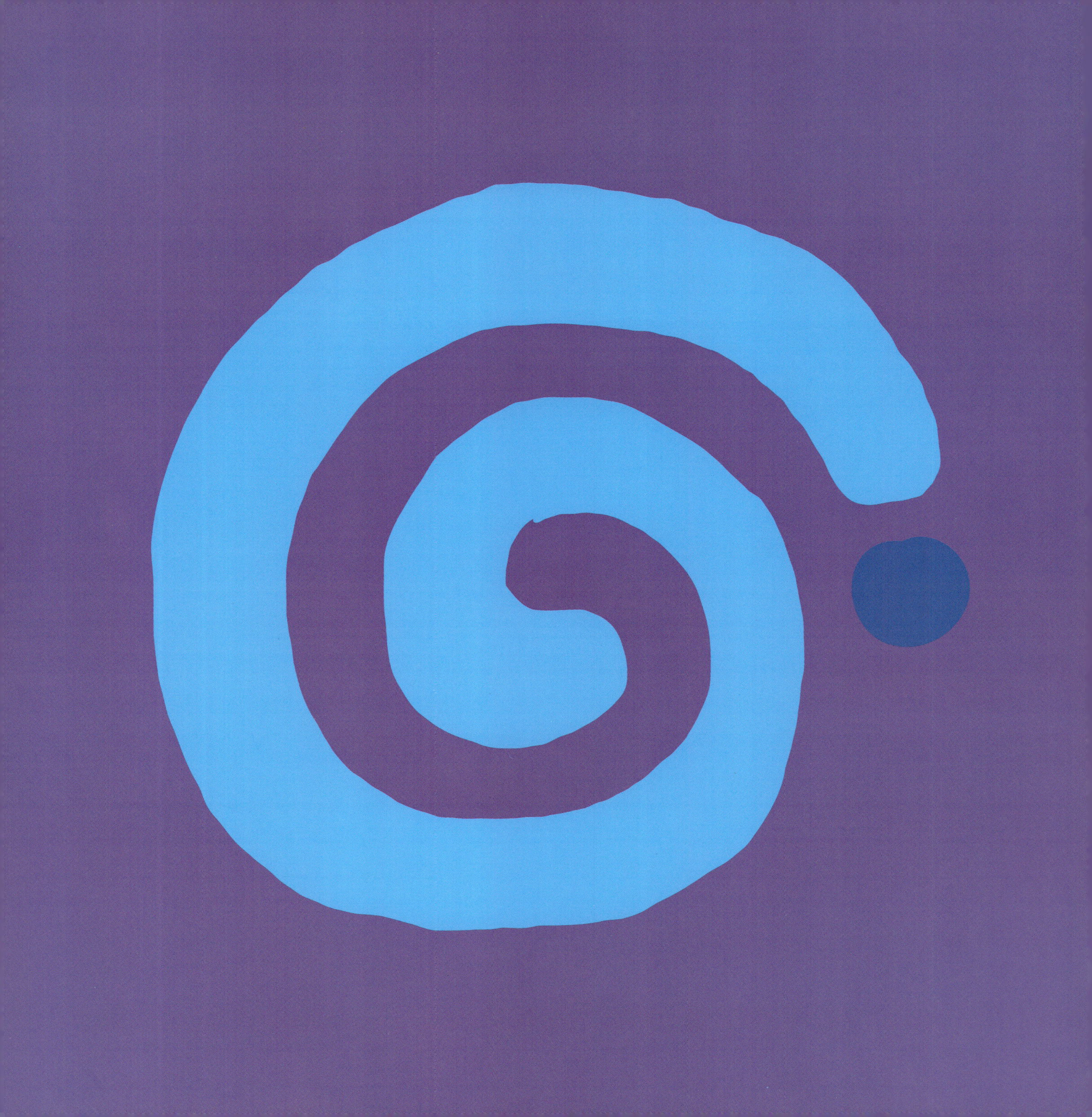

Pattern 34

With practise you can learn to recognise your thought patterns and find easier ways to encourage the good ones and interrupt the bad ones.

Thoughts are only thoughts, until you give an importance to them they will simply remain something harmless that comes and goes in your head. It isn't until we attribute importance to them that they can feel more real. Knowing this allows you to filter the negative or unimportant ones and reinforce those you want to keep thinking about.

The next time you start thinking about a subject you know could lead to darker areas, ask yourself 'Where did this thought start' or ask yourself 'What can I do to interrupt this thought?' Perhaps look at doing something differently to prevent the pattern recurring, **a simple act of intervention** such as standing up or going for a walk, can interrupt your spiralling thoughts if you were sat down.

Keeping a healthy view and understanding of your thoughts and thinking is a vital part of maintaining good mental health. The reassurance that you can spot and ultimately manage your patterns will add to your confidence.

"By recognising recurring patterns in your thinking and by identifying start points and triggers, you have the means to change them." Anon.

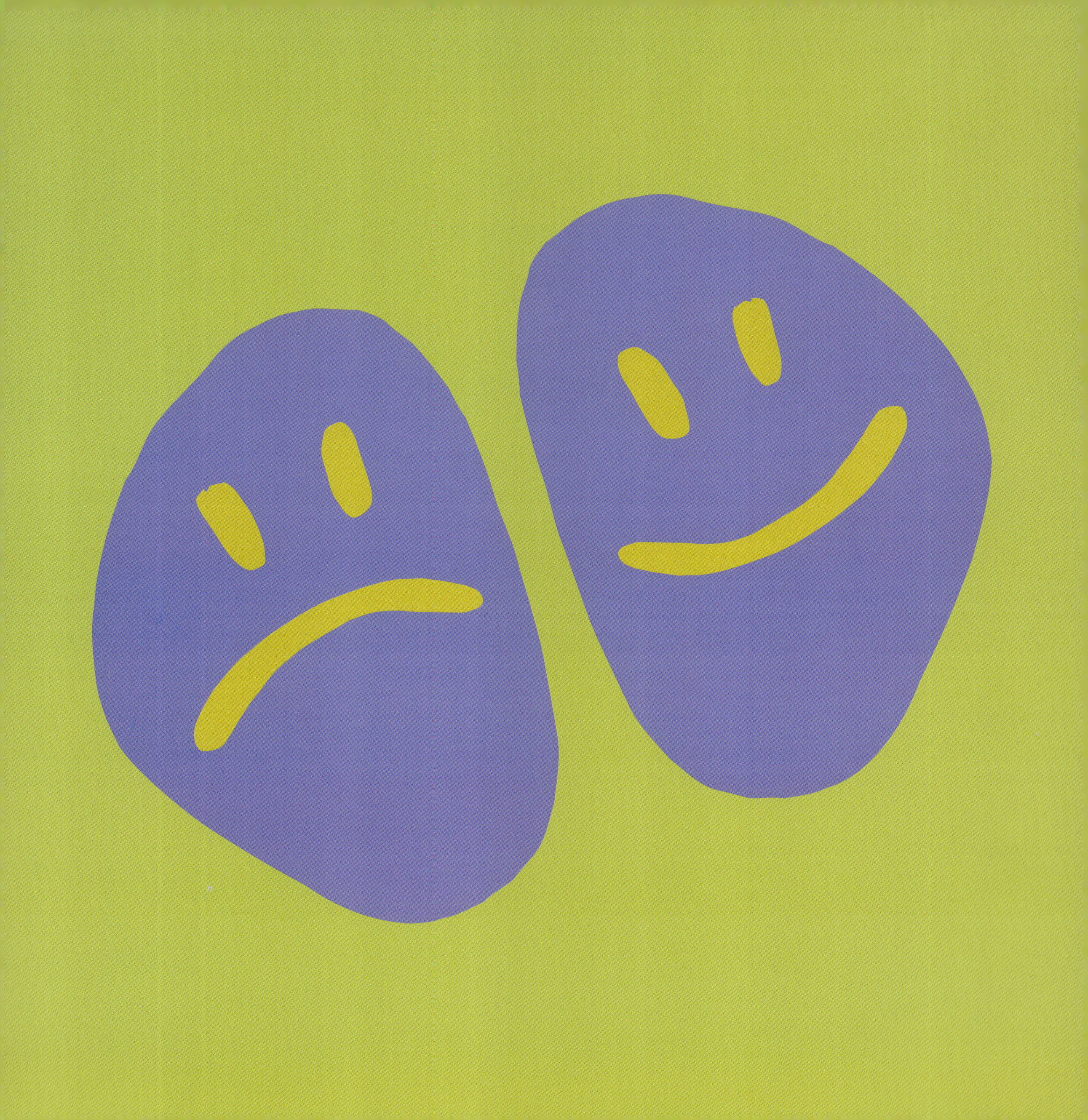

Attitude 35

Your thoughts can become internal feelings, which can in turn become expressions seen by others, positive or negative. Building a self confident internal you is key.

Simply approaching your day with a positive mindset may lead to feeling happy as your mood affects those around you. Smiling within yourself and thinking yourself into a positive mindset radiates through small, often imperceptible body language and expressions as well as larger and more obvious ones. Self-fulfilling prophesies can start with a thought.

Experiment: Try walking down the street feeling and looking grumpy with a negative expression. Count the number of smiles you get back. Then try the same walk with a smile and a determination to spread good cheer.

Practising control of your thoughts and attributing weight to the good ones helps encourage **a positive mindset**. Knowing yourself, your mind and an internal confidence is the foundation of a good or healthy outgoing attitude which encourages good responses in others.

"Your living is determined not so much by what life brings to you as by the attitude you bring to life; not so much by what happens to you as by the way your mind looks at what happens. Khalil Gibran

"Attitude is a little thing that makes a big difference. Winston Churchill

“You are in control of your own thoughts”

**“Positive thoughts
lead to
positive feelings
which
leads to a
positive mood.”**

5 Summary

Key to finding your most positive attitude is an open mindedness to learn and ask questions. Accepting the differences of others improves your life overall.

Finding a good mindset will be quickly reinforced by the people around you. They will see the difference and behave differently.

By taking a positive approach to problems, regardless of your situation, you will soon find a better world for yourself.

Patience and a determination to spot your mind habits can eventually give you the control you want to add to your bank of wellbeing, safe in the knowledge you are the best you can be on the inside. But be kind to yourself, the mind is a seriously complex organ and takes some understanding.

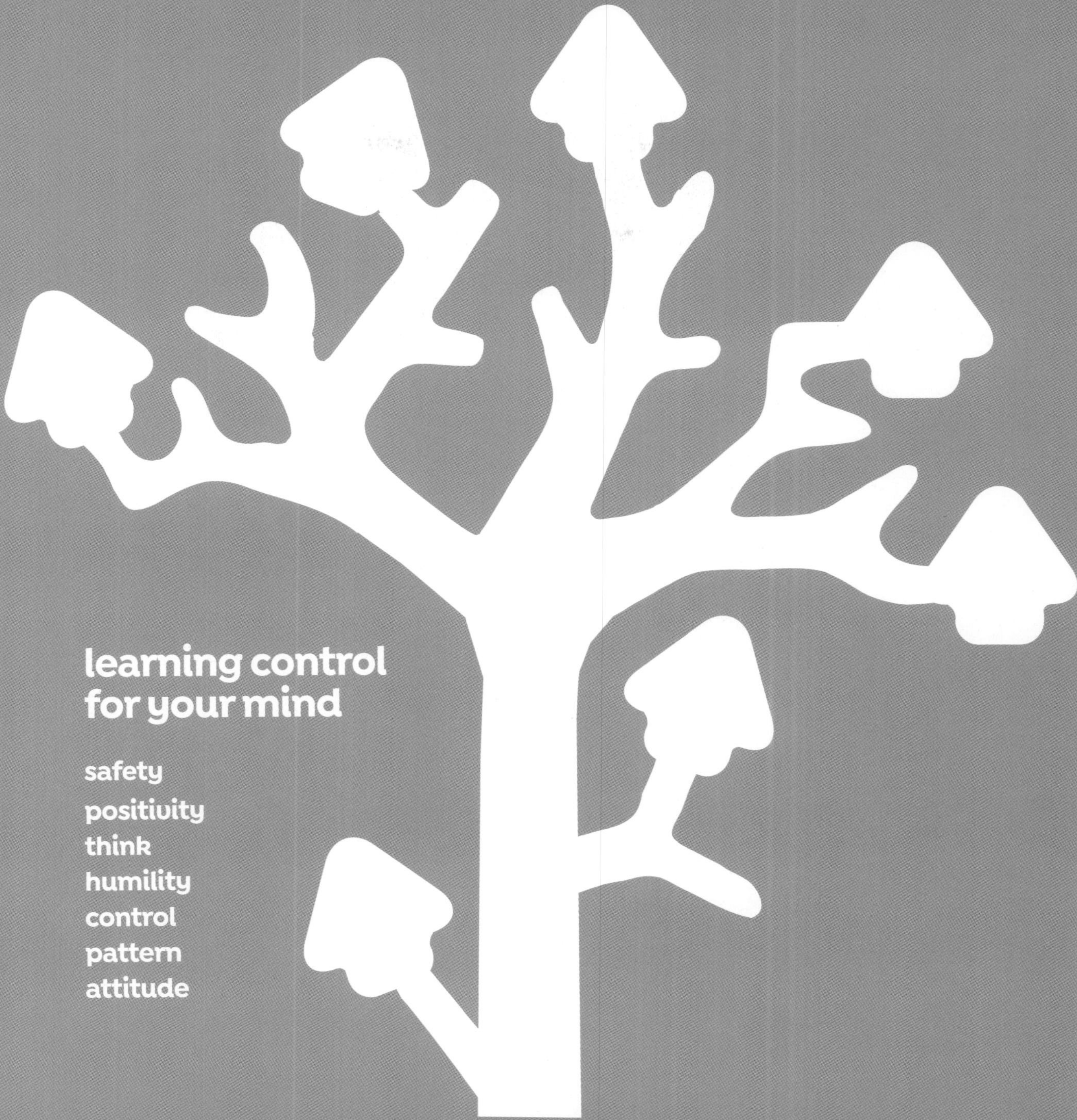

learning control for your mind

safety
positivity
think
humility
control
pattern
attitude

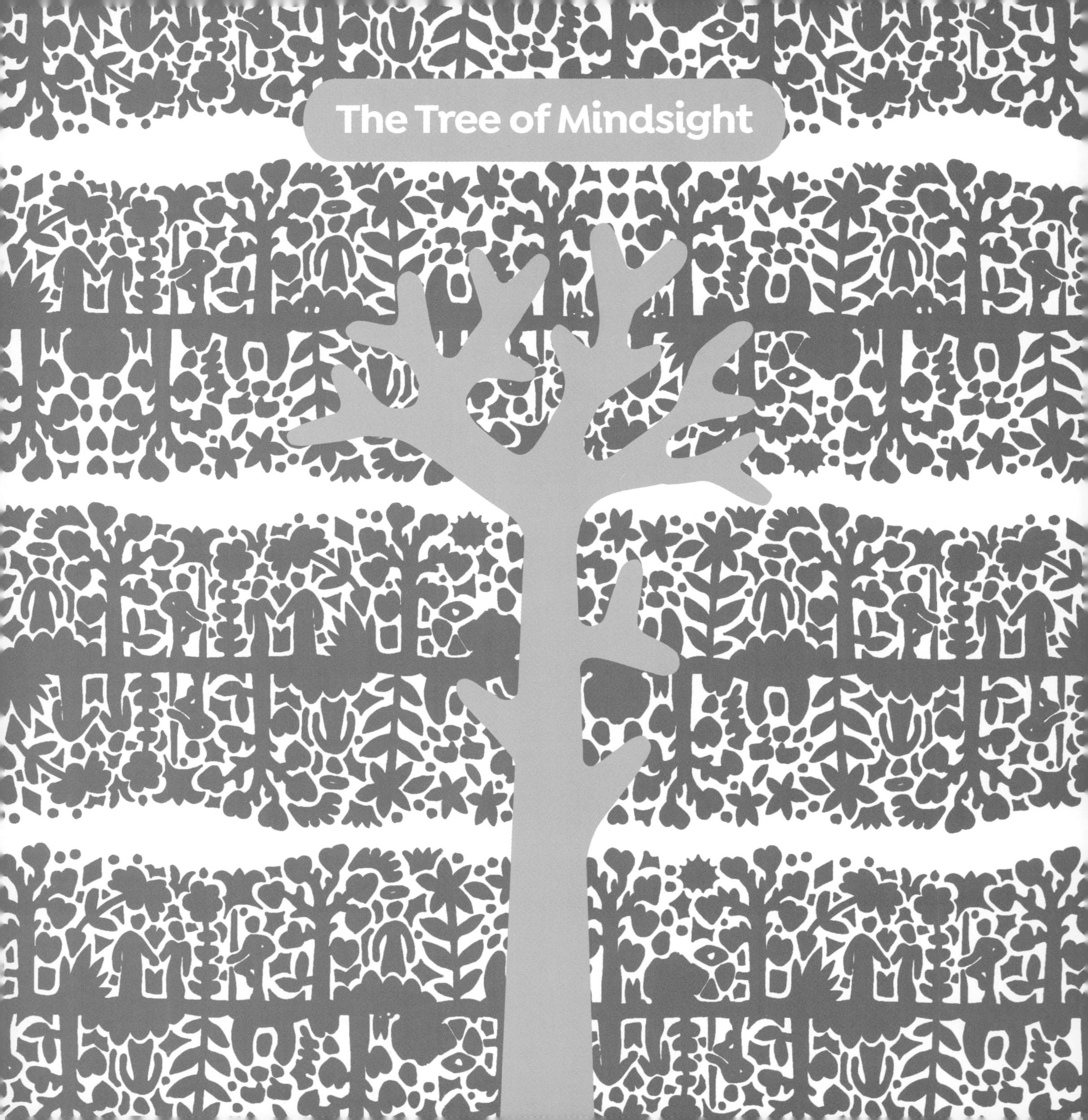
The Tree of Mindsight

6

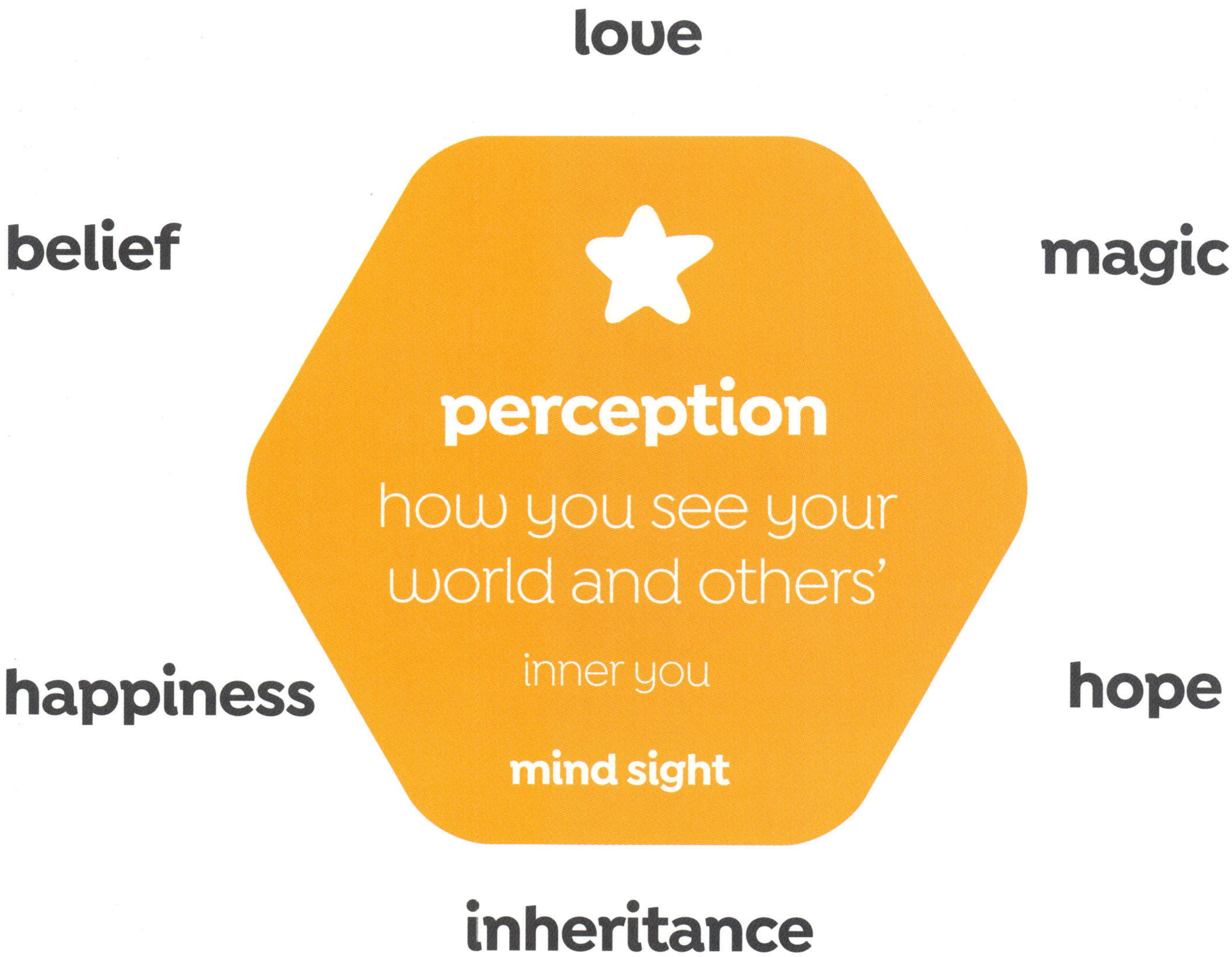
love
belief
magic
perception
how you see your world and others'
inner you
mind sight
happiness
hope
inheritance

6 Your Mindsight

The sixth tree is the tree of mindsight, it is all about understanding perception, how you see yourself and other people's lives.

By understanding how you see both your past and current influences, what is inherited and how your beliefs can flex, you can build a stronger picture of the self you wish to be. Finding a better love for yourself can allow others to love you too, with mutual growth building a more joyful and happy world of better wellbeing. In this system this is called mindsight, the way these viewpoints shape your perception of yourself and others.

The following questions, quotes and insights are a summary of the essential elements that help you see yourself and your world, one keyword at a time.

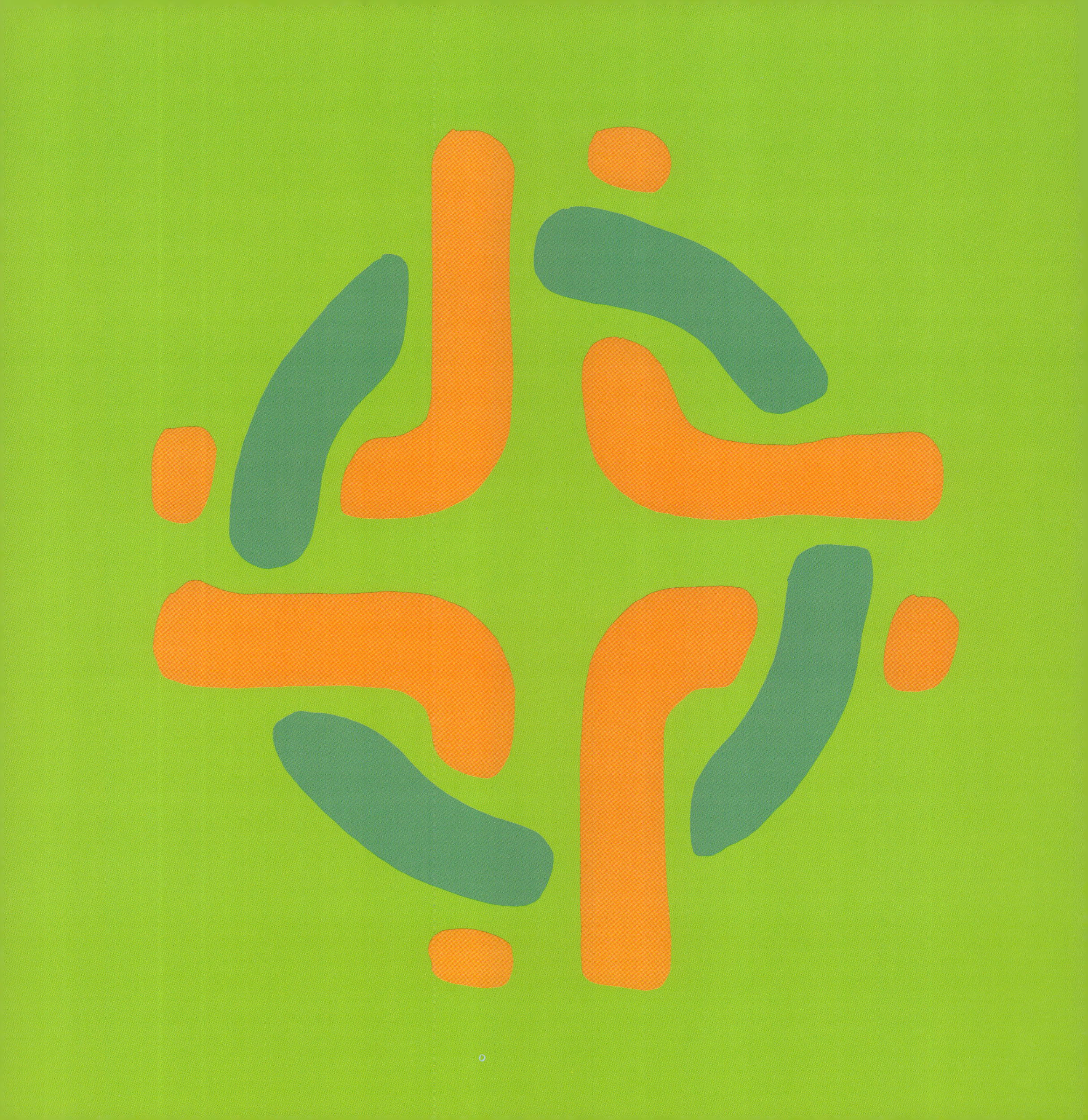

Belief

36

Often all that stands in our way of achieving our goal is the simple belief that we can't. Self belief is key.

Beliefs can be challenged, questioned and ultimately adjusted for self-improvement. They may be different from our values, which we may inherit, and are treasured firmly held foundation stones of ourselves.

Ask yourself, 'Where do my beliefs come from?', 'Are they my own or have I inherited them?', 'What do I really believe in?', '**What is a belief that I CAN change to make my life better**, and what is a value to me that I am unlikely to change?'

Understanding your beliefs and values allows you to assess what you really believe in and with practise allow yourself to filter and change if you want to. By understanding which are your beliefs and opinions and which are somebody else's, you can develop a stronger sense of who you are, and similarly a better understanding of others.

"Enlightened leadership is spiritual if we understand spirituality not as some kind of religious dogma or ideology but as the domain of awareness where we experience values like truth, goodness, beauty, love and compassion, and also intuition, creativity, insight and focused attention." Deepak Chopra

Magic

Aim to achieve a state of living magically, even in everyday life. It pays to shoot for the moon, if you miss you might hit the stars.

Living magically is a wonderful way of seeing the world positively. This approach can lift you both beautifully and naturally out and above everyday mundane lives. It is a lifestyle choice that involves shooting for the moon, believing we can reach for a higher goal.

Ask yourself, 'What is actually stopping me from doing something?' Often the answers will reveal hurdles that can be overcome, so keep asking and finding your own answers until you find the truth.

The benefits of reaching or achieving something you previously thought unachievable are a fabulous addition to your overall bank of general wellbeing. The process of achieving this and finding the true obstacles that lie in the way, in your head or otherwise, are always going to be a great lift. One could say it is magic.

"I am a great admirer of mystery and magic. Look at this life – all mystery and magic." Harry Houdini

"And above all, watch with glittering eyes the whole world around you because the greatest secrets are always hidden in the most unlikely places. Those who don't believe in magic will never find it." Roald Dahl

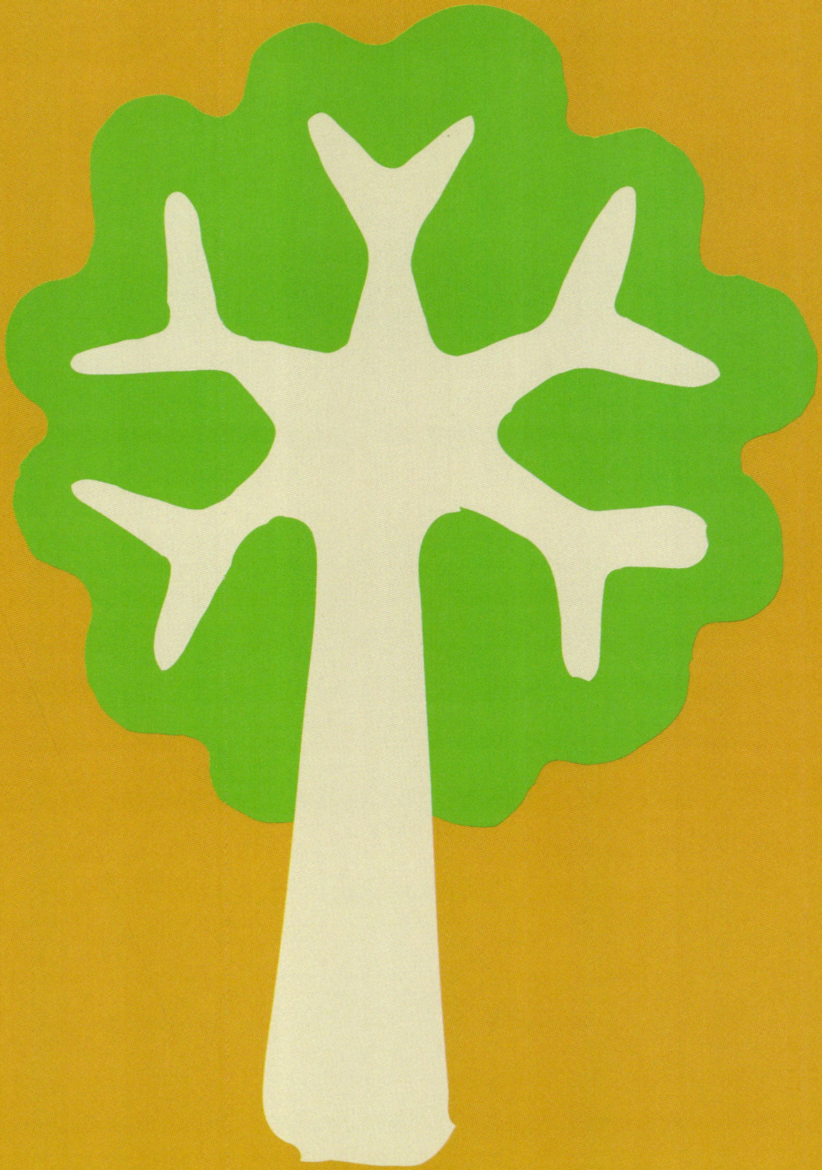

★ Inheritance 38

The way we see ourselves is a product of what we have inherited, through experience and genetically, and what we choose to be.

Who you are and who you see yourself as, are made up of the three elements - your past experiences, what you were born with and what you decide to be in the future. Inheritance, for the purposes of this book is all our past experiences. It is the memories we acquire as we travel through the forest of life, and the characteristics we live with which we inherited. These elements define who we see ourselves as, our solid selves, and sometimes how we behave.

'**How much of my past has affected who I am**, and how can I learn to understand this. How do I accept this and how do I fit this information and these lessons from my past into my today?'

What has happened to us affects the way we think about our current selves, understanding this will lead to our truth. We need to accept the honest picture of who we were, our past selves, our inheritance both genetically and experientially. This acceptance is then key to moving forward with more confidence and living more easily with ourselves into the future.

"Genetics do play a role in how you consciously or subconsciously manifest your true self." Ben Harper

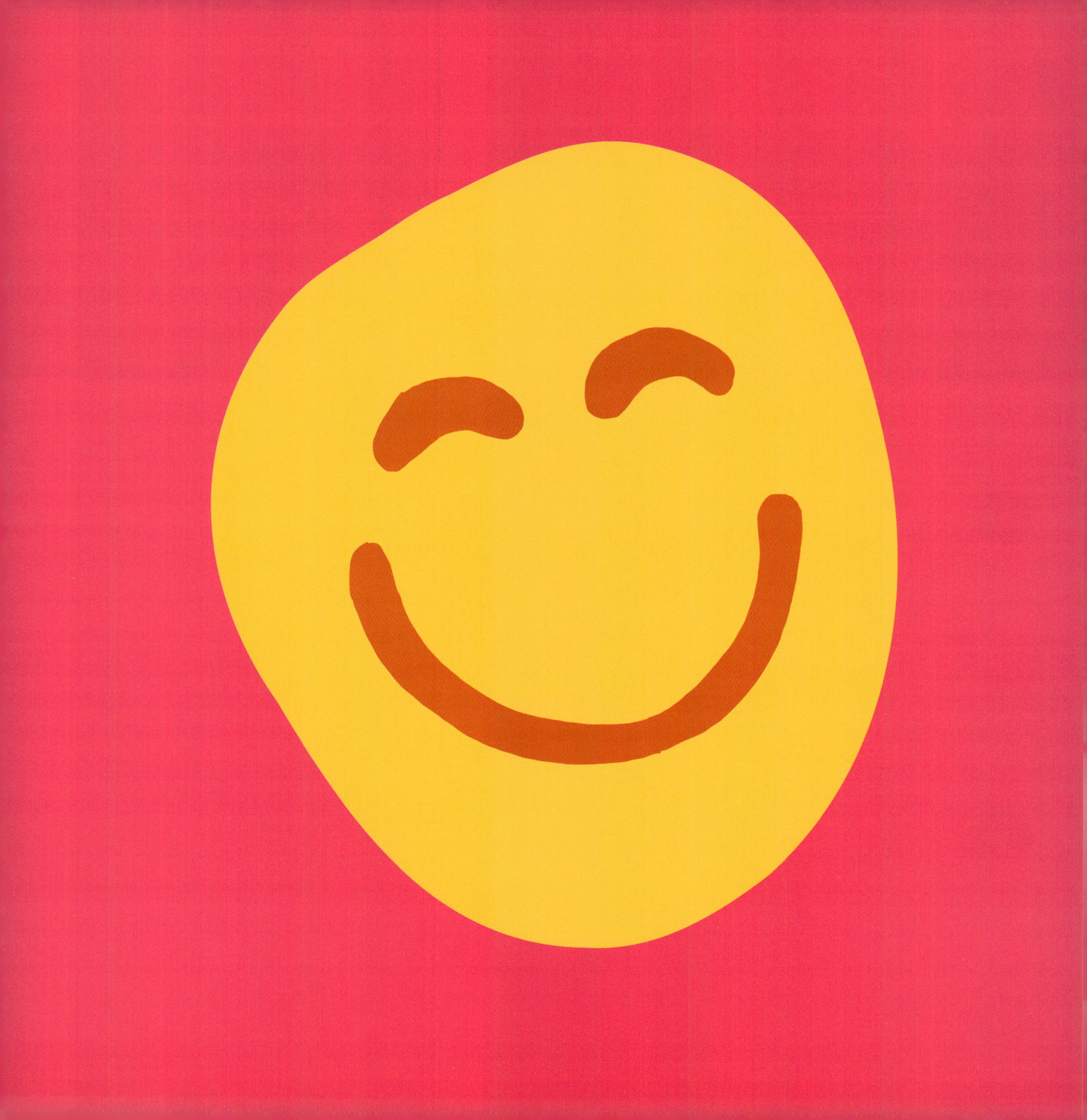

★ Happiness 39

Happiness is a state of mind, it doesn't have to be dependent on anything. You can decide to be happy anytime. Woo Hoo!

The hardest part of the journey to personal happiness is investing the time. Time to learn to understand you are in control of your happiness, time to unpick the perceived hurdles, some seemingly impossible, challenge them and then see them differently.

A great question to keep asking yourself is 'Will spending this time have a long lasting effect on my happiness?' Invest in your happiness or will it may only be a short term pleasure, soon forgotten.

If you look at happiness as a life of good experiences, then adding to this by taking actions with a long term positive benefit is a great strategy for a strong overall foundation of wellbeing. **The best time spent is so often with other people***, friends, family, groups or even strangers, giving, sharing and joyously celebrating life in places like football matches, concerts or occasional mountain tops. That said, brief memorable experiences such as dancing, giggling, singing and laughing can add to the long term bank of happiness in your life too! *Note: Some of us are introverts who find great happiness with ourselves!

"If you want others to be happy, practice compassion. If you want to be happy, practice compassion. Happiness is not something ready made. It comes from your own actions. Dalai Lama

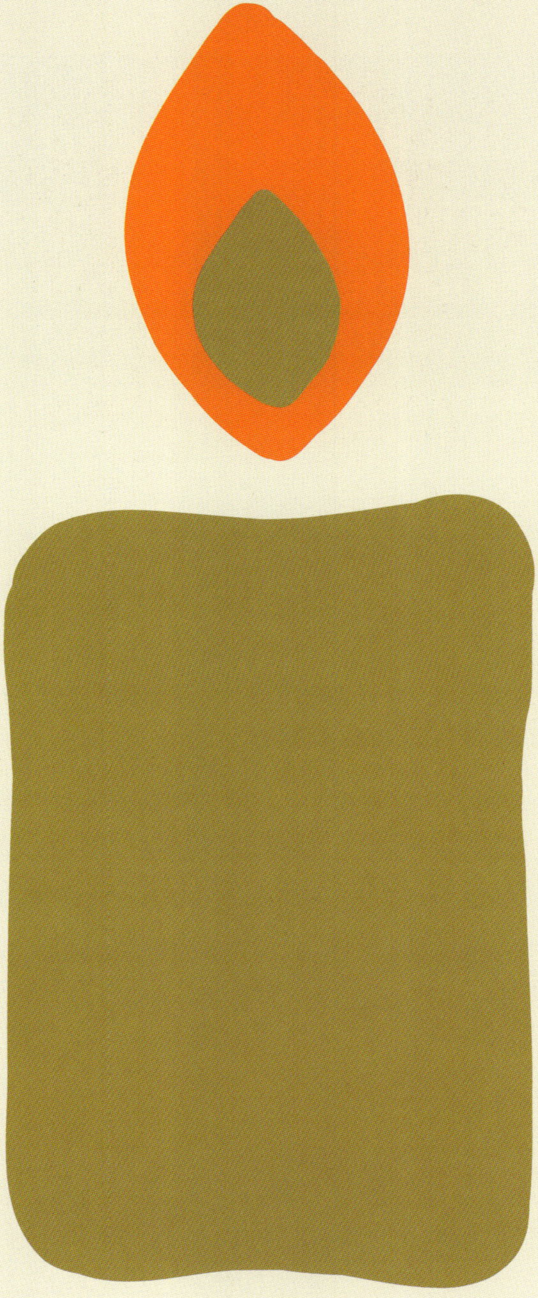

★ Hope 40

Hope drives you to your future vision of yourself, it is the motivational force. When all of the comfort of our lives is stripped away, it is the last resort for a better life.

It is easy to lose hope and your drive, it is far harder to create the forces that pull you to a brighter future. These forces are the positivity, the drive and motivation behind all your actions, the light at the end of the tunnel and your vision of your future self.

Ask yourself 'How do I see myself in five year's time?', 'What do I look like, what do I think about my life. Is this future me positive, am I happy, do I have many friends and if so what do they look like?' Paint yourself a picture of your future self and try working backwards from that.

The benefits of understanding and embracing hope for your future wellbeing are everywhere to be seen and all embracing.
Hope is essential to get you to your end destination, regardless.

"Hope is the thing with feathers that perches in the soul - and sings the tunes without the words - and never stops at all." Emily Dickinson

"We must accept finite disappointment, but never lose infinite hope." Martin Luther King

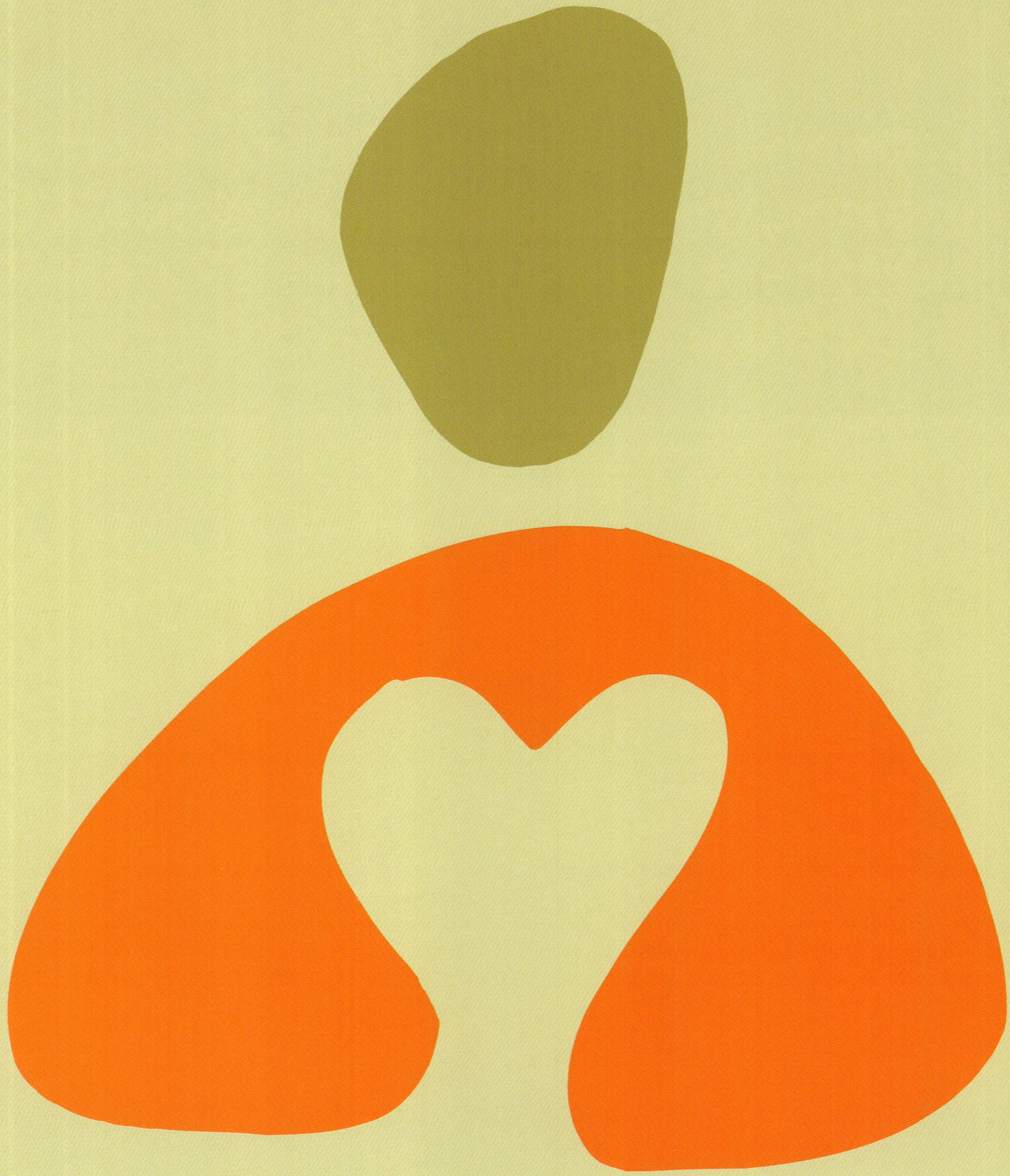

★ Love (of self) 41

Learning to love living with your self and with your mind, understanding how it works and how you see you and those around you in the world, is a beautiful warm goal.

Loving yourself starts with an understanding and acceptance of how you see yourself and the world in general. Then it is through action and interaction with others that we see a better us doing good in the world and find this **marvellous inner warmth.**

Asking yourself, 'What do you see when you see you?' will probably take you down a long road of further questioning. Unpicking these answers will reveal certain aspects of yourself. The truth of you is never easy, but every difficulty overcome builds a better and stronger you.

Developing this self-knowledge and being honest with yourself at all times leads you to the ultimate goal of **'I like me'.** How you see yourself and finding this place could be a reflection of yourself in other people's lives. It is a warm and magnetic place once you start down this road.

"Trust yourself. Create the kind of self that you will be happy to live with all your life. Make the most of yourself by fanning the tiny, inner sparks of possibility into flames of achievement." Golda Meir

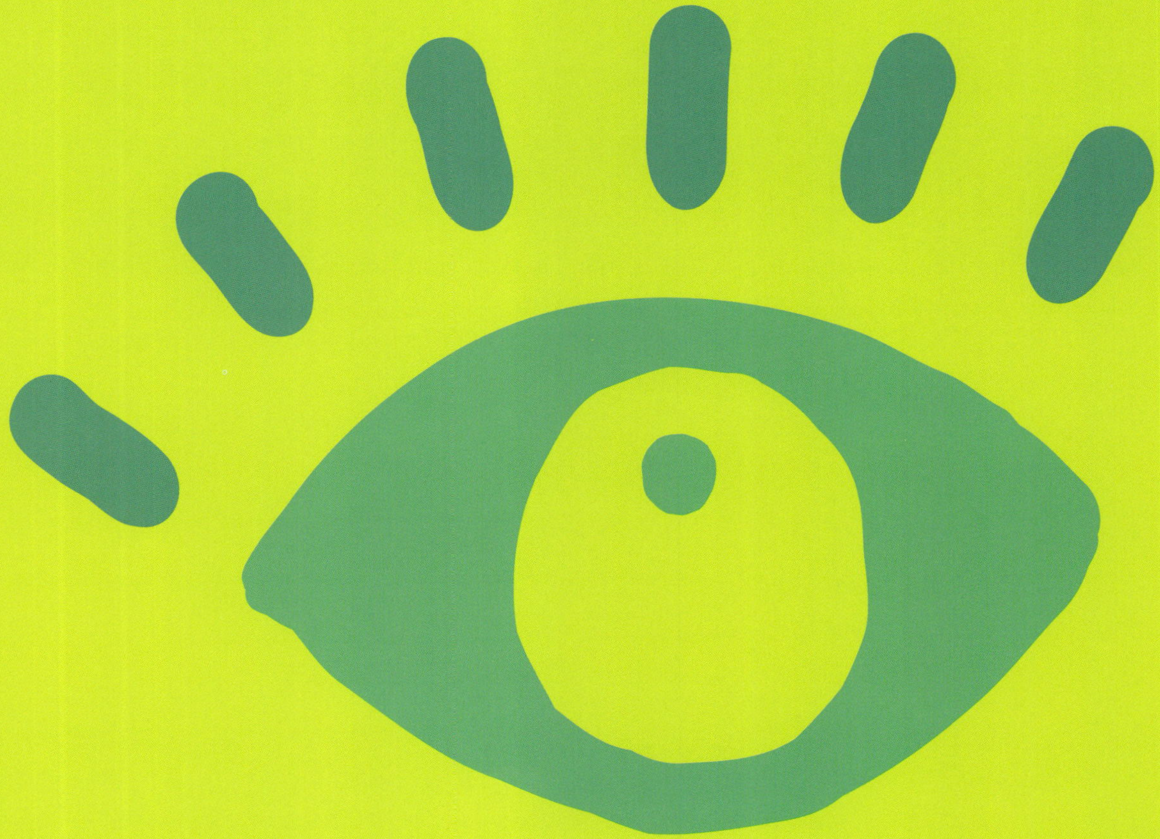

★ Perception 42

We all have the power to control how we interpret how we 'see' ourselves, other people and the world.

What is important here is to understand the concept that **we all 'see' things differently** and that we put our own 'take' on how we 'see' things, people, the world and how the world 'sees' us. This is perception.

Ask yourself next time you strenuously disagree with someone, 'Would I feel differently about this person if I could see the world through their eyes?' Ask yourself, 'What experiences they may have been through to be like this?' and then, 'do I now appreciate this and feel differently towards them?'

The challenge is understanding and appreciating your own viewpoint and its many influences, then learning to 'see' the world through somebody else's eyes. This is hard, as there will be many unknown factors affecting how they 'see' things, but the act of trying is truly educating. A greater **respect for the viewpoints of other people** means you see others in a better light and in turn this respect is often reciprocated. It is core for your mindsight and helps build your solid foundation of wellbeing.

"What you see is not what others see. We inhabit parallel worlds of perception, bounded by our interests and experience. What is obvious to some is invisible to others." George Monbiot

"How you see yourself and how you see the world is a choice you are in control of."

"It is important to question your beliefs, and more importantly, whether they are truly yours."

6 Summary

You are who you see yourself as. You are in control of this so it makes sense to ask how and why you see yourself as you do.

Finding a spark of appreciation for who you are, what you have done in this world and the warmth that follows is a worthy goal.

The road that you need to follow to achieve this love of yourself starts with a need for you to see you for you, others for who they are and the world in general. This is not going to be easy but you can do it respectfully, joyously and happily if you decide to. It will help you and build your best wellbeing.

Discovering that the vast majority of us are kind, loving and compassionate is more than enough motivation. It is a warm feeling.

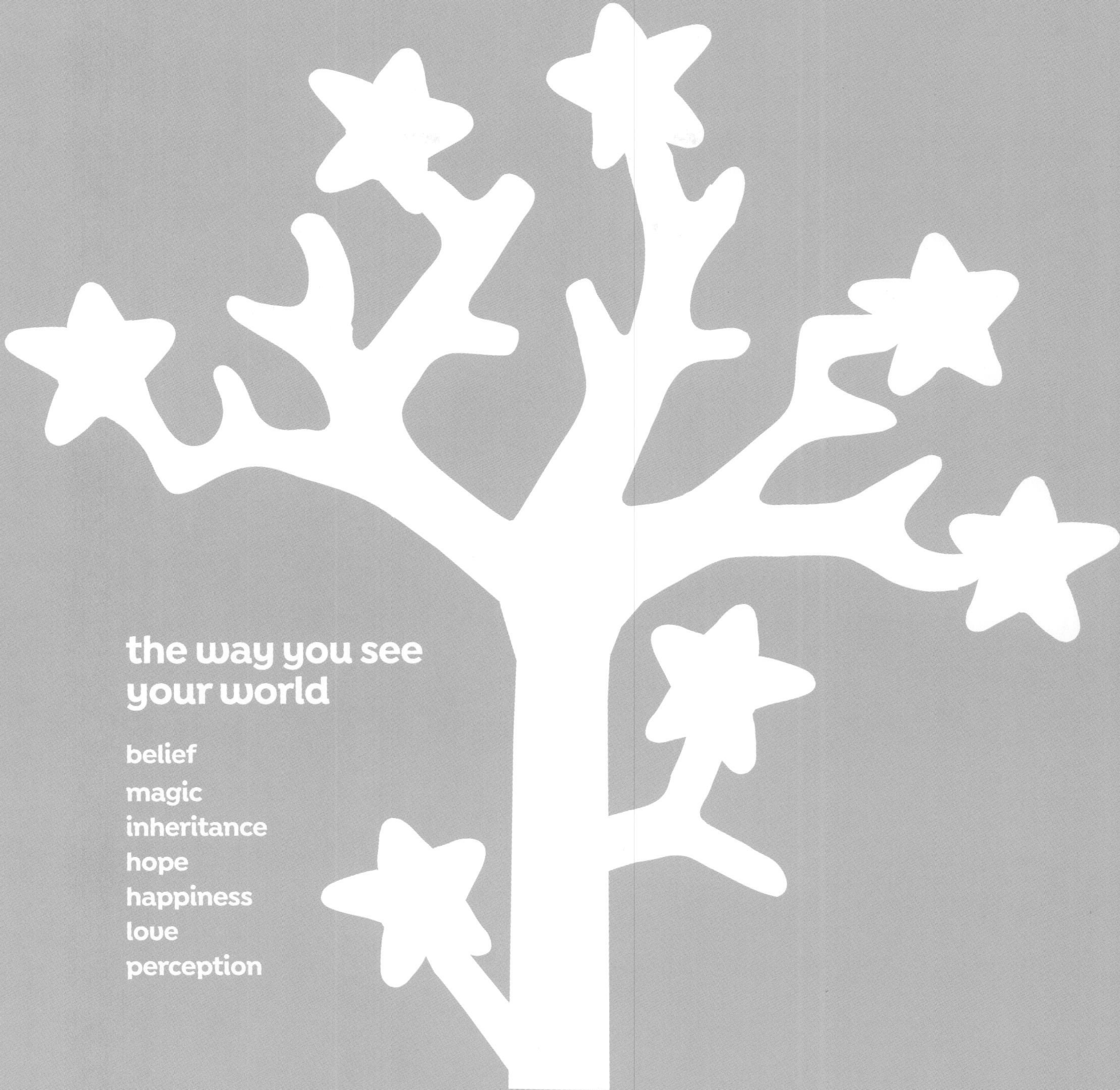

the way you see your world

belief
magic
inheritance
hope
happiness
love
perception

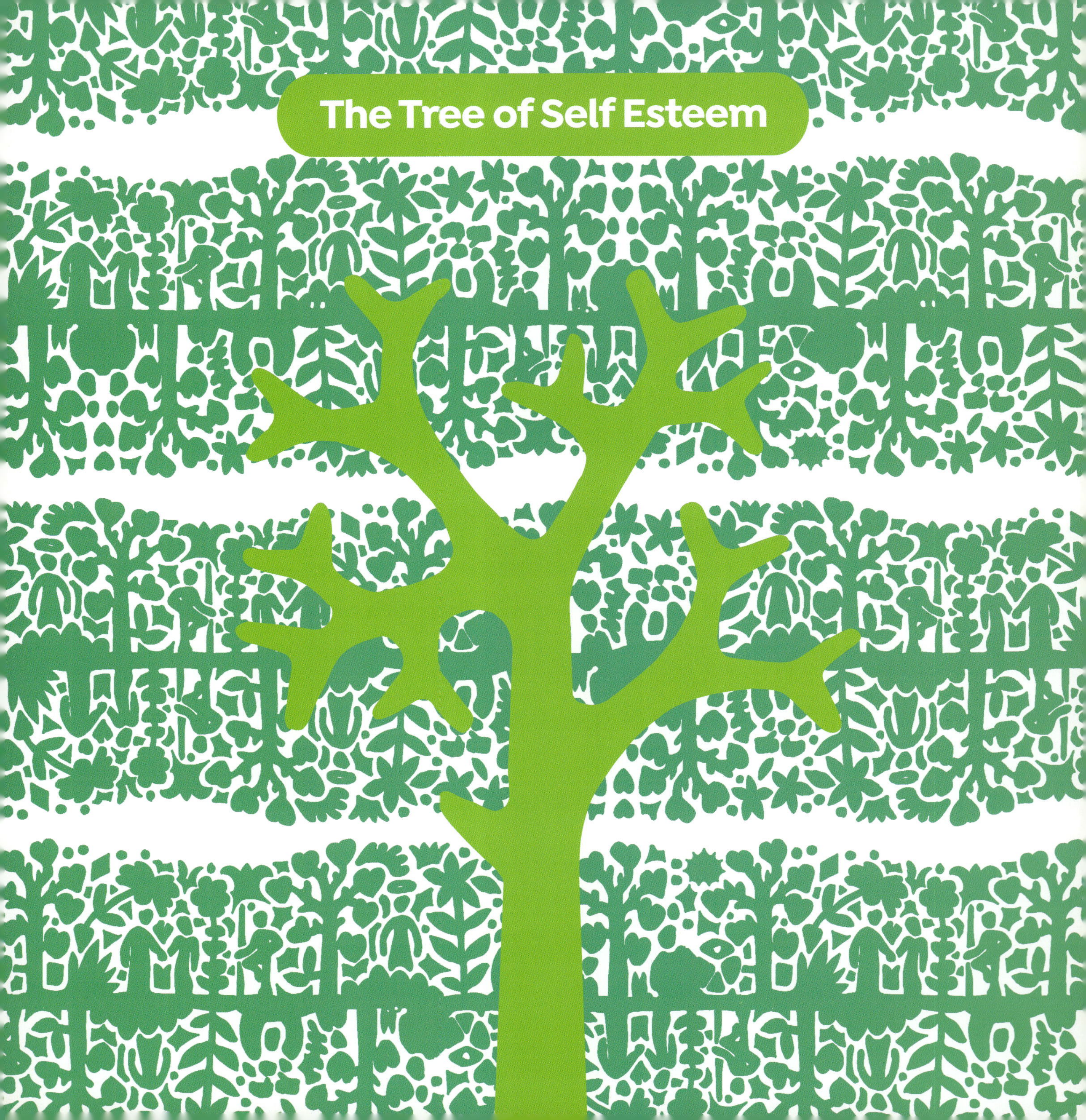
The Tree of Self Esteem

7

kindness

empathy

bravery

confidence

building your self esteem.

interface you

mind work

giving

sharing

tolerance

7 Your Self Esteem

The Tree of Self Esteem is the seventh tree in the Magic Forest, it is all about building your self esteem through interaction.

These words are about the way your actions and behaviour interface with your world – 'Actions that can speak louder than thoughts'.

By taking your thoughts and respectfully turning them into interaction with others in your life, you can add to your overall strength of personal wellbeing through kindness, empathy, sharing, giving, bravery and tolerance... building your confidence by building mutual respect from others.

The following questions, quotes and insights are a summary of the essential elements to help you start building your self esteem, one action or one deed at a time.

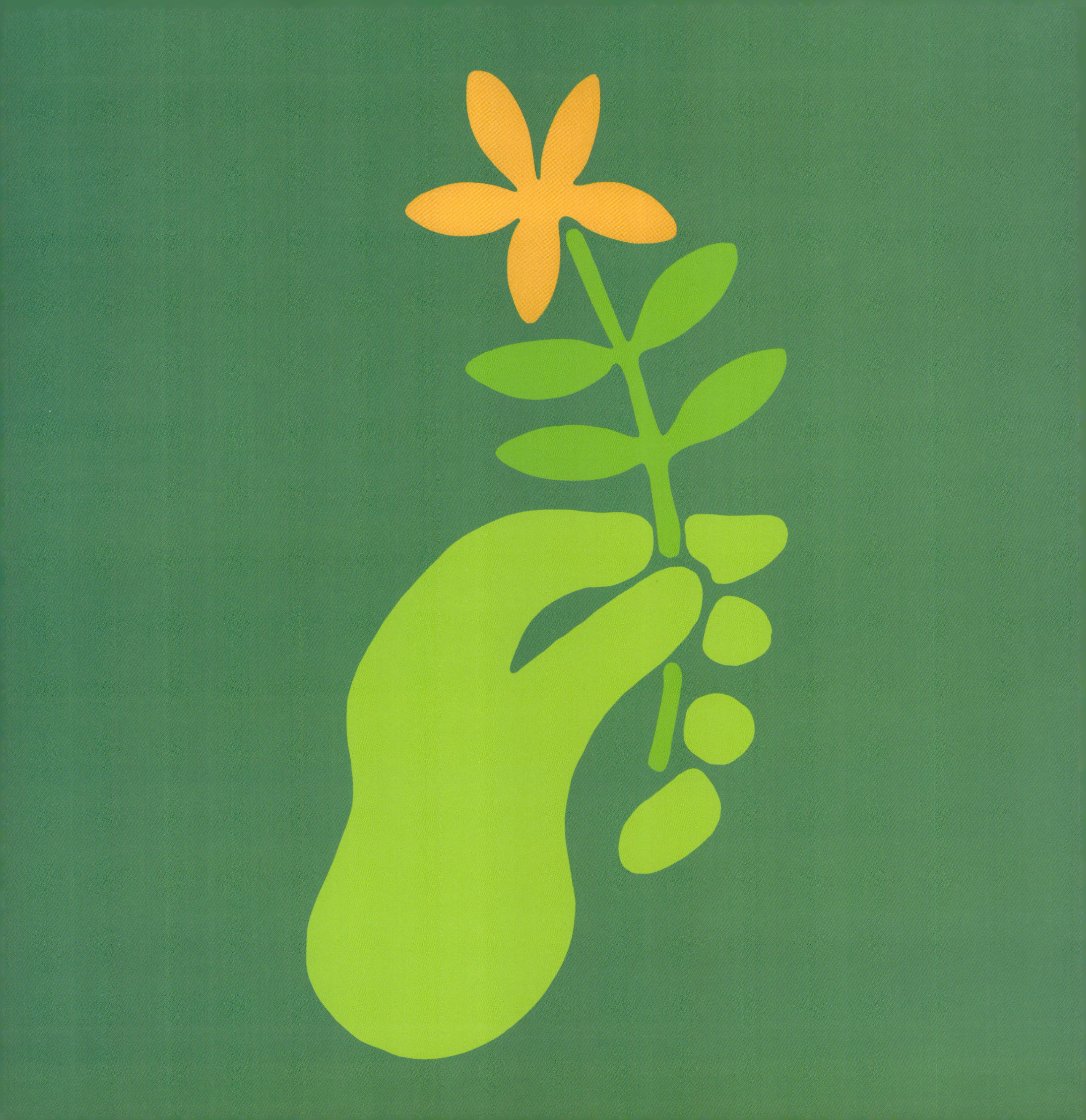

✚ Kindness 43

Kindness is the most human action, where considerate thoughts turn to generous acts through friendly hands.

A kindness can be the simplest thing to you and might make a massive difference to someone in need. There is a movement worthy of more inspection, founded on the belief that acts of kindness can lead to more kind acts in the future, 'Paying it Forward'.

You could challenge yourself to carry out a **random act of kindness.** Seeking no reward, do something for somebody else, perhaps in an unexpected way or anonymously, without being asked. The results are disproportionately rewarding and sometimes unexpected.

The good deeds you do, however small, from a smile to full blown philanthropy, Bill Gates style, can lead to a greater consideration for others, a better understanding of yourself and an overall increased self esteem. Not only is **a world full of kindness** a much more considerate, fun, thoughtful and caring environment for everyone to grow up and live in but the simple acts that you carry out make you feel great.

"Too often we underestimate the power of a touch, a smile, a kind word, a listening ear, an honest compliment, or the smallest act of caring, all of which have the potential to turn a life around."
Leo Buscaglia

Empathy 44

This first step in understanding others puts yourself in somebody else's shoes and allows you to see your world as well as theirs.

Put simply empathy is the ability to **understand and share feelings** for another. There is cognitive and affective empathy to think about.

The challenging question to answer to gain an understanding of other people's beliefs, opinions, values and life choices is to ask yourself, 'How would I feel if I were living as that person in their situation?'

By seeing the world through other people's eyes, a fresh viewpoint, you broaden your understanding of the vast range of different feelings and experiences we all live through. Stripped away from material trappings, we all reduce to our core human feelings and relationships. The truth of all of us. It shows us **how similar we all are in our life** ambitions, cares and worries. The feelings inherited through empathy for others quickly broadens the width of your own shoulders and can give you more twinkly, caring eyes.

"In my view, the best of humanity is in our exercise of empathy and compassion. It's when we challenge ourselves to walk in the shoes of someone whose pain or plight might seem so different than yours that it's almost incomprehensible". Sarah McBride

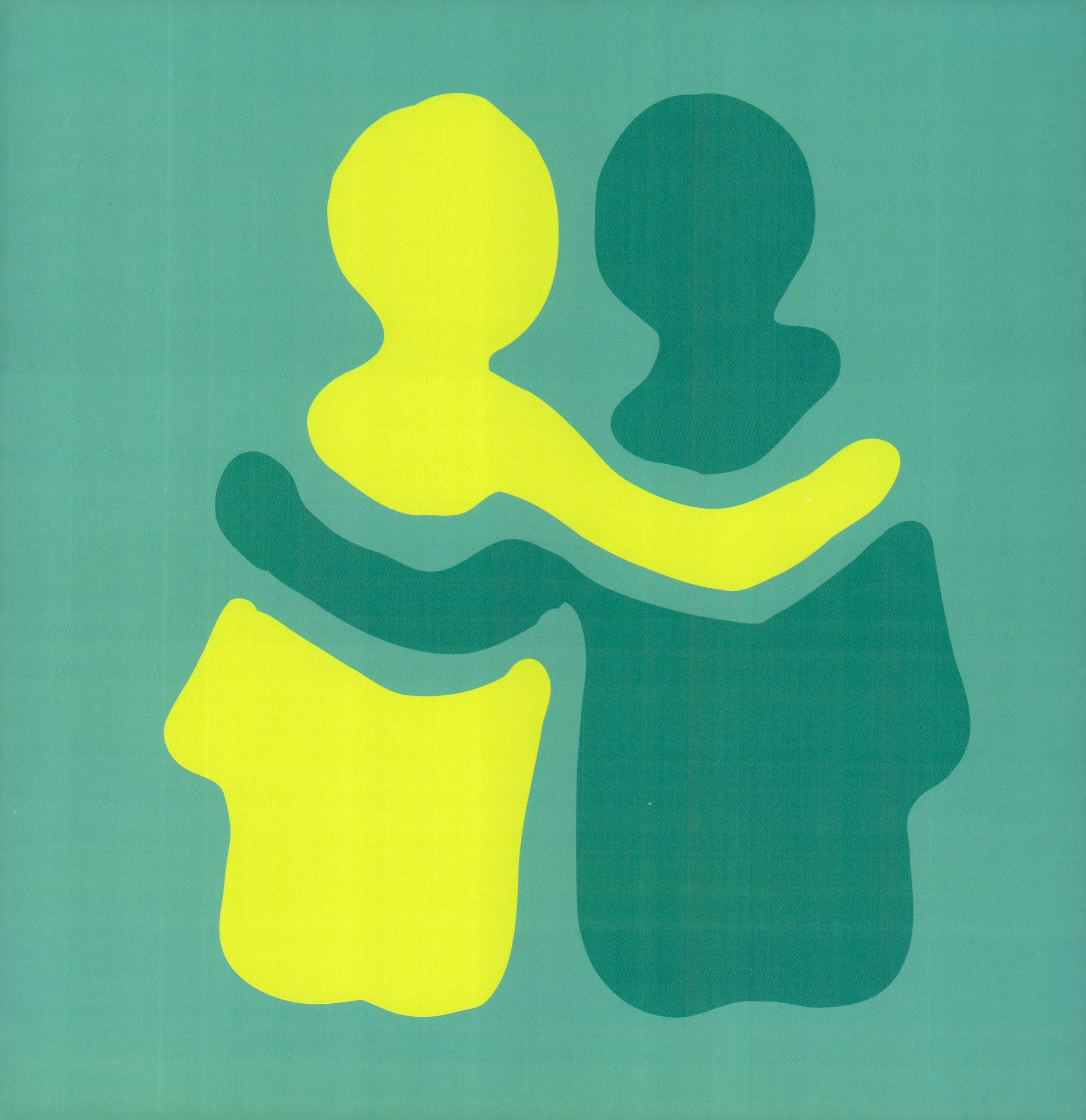

Sharing 45

By sharing thoughts, feelings and our everyday life we broaden our relationships and strengthen our personal confidence.

By sharing we learn to work together, our communication improves, our experiences are shared, and our lives are all the richer for it. As with all great truths, sharing is no different. Learning to accept the truth that **we are all flawed** and that we all have differences born of our own experiences, makes us stronger through acceptance and most importantly through learning to share them and living together.

Try extending conversations beyond pleasantries and asking sincerely interested questions in a friend. Try asking 'How are you doing right now?' and wait for the answer. It's surprisingly rare.

Accepting that everyone has something to give, everyone has experiences that have flawed them, however seemingly great the apparent differences, **we can always learn something from everyone.** Nobody is perfect and accepting this for yourself is a first step on the path to a more confident and fearless you.

"*There is no joy in possession without sharing.*" Erasmus

"*The miracle is this: The more we share the more we have.*" Leonard Nimoy

"*The fundamental law of human beings is interdependence. A person is a person through other persons.*" Archbishop Desmond Tutu

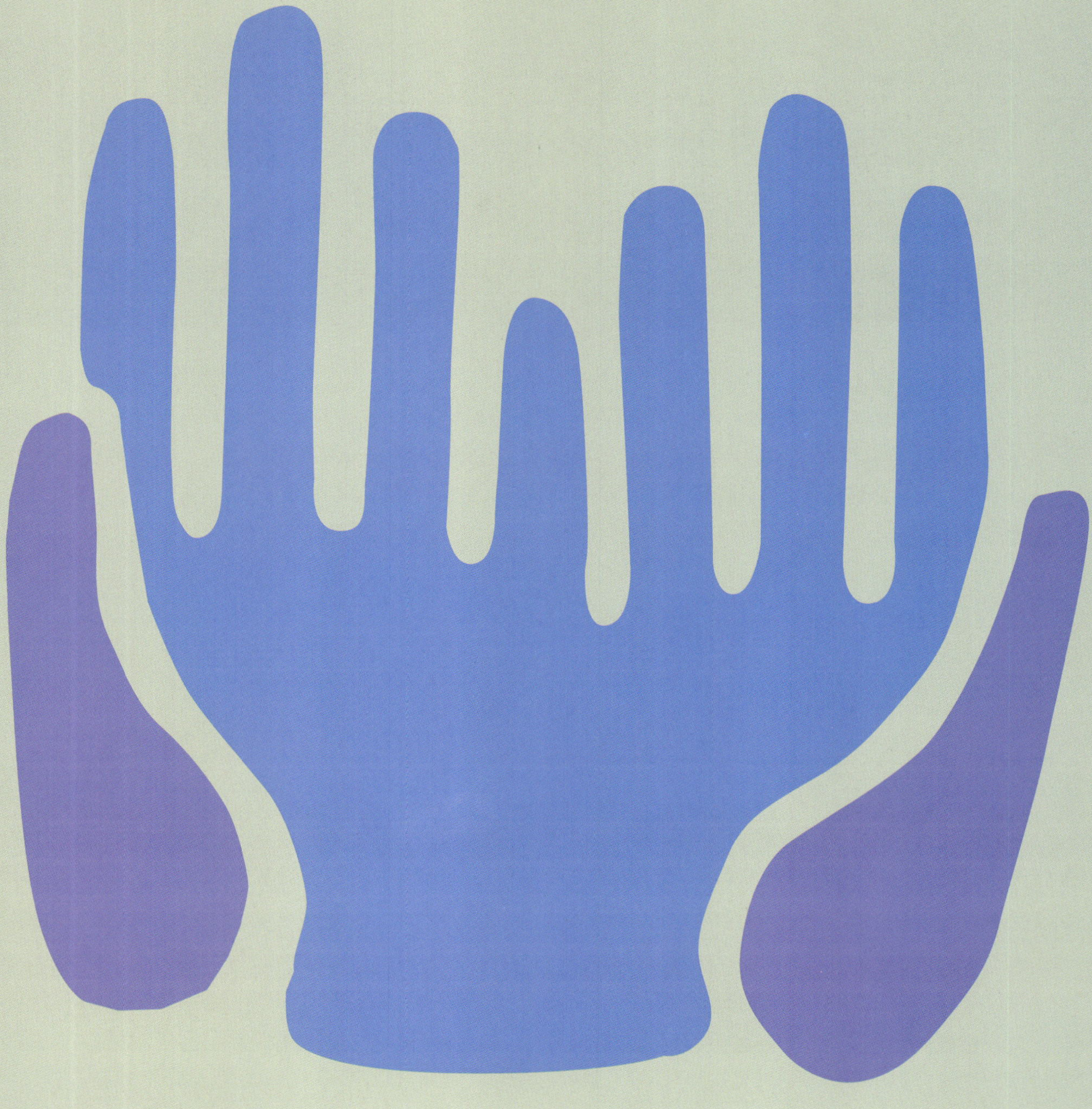

✚ Giving 46

Giving can be emotional, a smile, a wave, a hug. It need not be material. Give a nod, give a pound but really give a care.

Giving is at the heart of finding the root level of your confidence in yourself and your ability to trust others to take without causing you hurt. Starting simply allows you to build this slowly. Giving your time as concentrated and sincere listening is a great way to start, costs nothing and could mean the earth to someone.

Try some small scale giving, a smile, or a hug with permission, always ask first. Give your time to someone once a day, if only for a few moments. Do this with an open mind, ready to listen, and you will find a wonderful rich seam of great stories to be mined.

Through giving, we learn to trust. Through trusting other people we can improve all our relations and in turn develop an understanding of others and an appreciation that we are not isolated and need not be alone. It all builds a more confident you.

"Give what you can without expectation. That is enough to make you the richest person on the planet." Anon

"My father said there were two kinds of people in the world: givers and takers. The takers may eat better, but the givers sleep better." Marlo Thomas

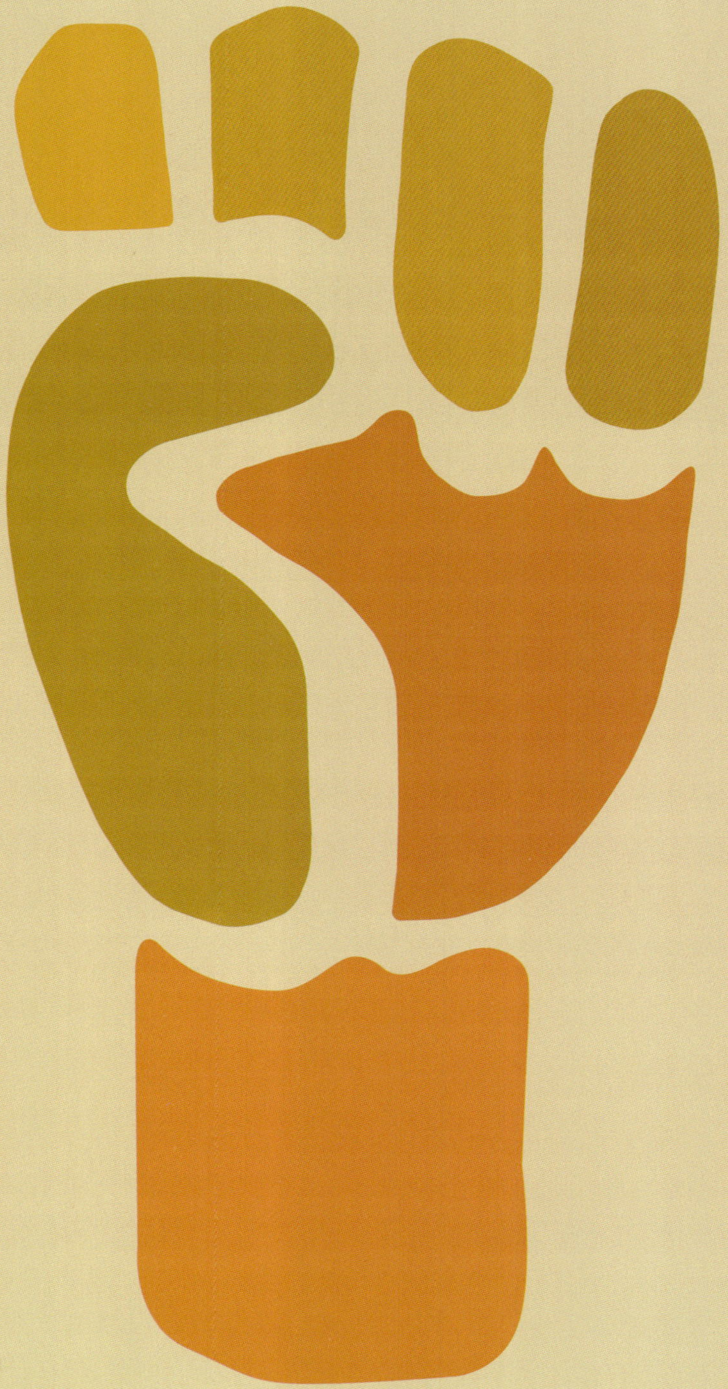

✚ Bravery 47

Finding the courage to get out of your comfort zone, with the possibility of failure, and then accepting the consequences will quickly build a more confident you.

The benefits and rewards of finding the courage to do something new, or change something, are usually disproportionate. Nearly everything you have done and are proud of will have started with an act of bravery that you might not have done had circumstances been different.

Try changing the way you approach a problem, try changing the way you see a relationship, or just try changing an everyday habit.
Ask yourself, 'What's really stopping me?' and work to understand the answer.

Trying to change and to do something new or differently is not easy. Without change there is going to be little personal growth. So you will need to try some courage to change. Whatever you choose to do, **get out of your comfort zone.** It has so many benefits you can't see.

"Fortune favours the brave" Anon

"Until one is committed, there is always hesitancy, the chance to draw back, always ineffectiveness. ...Whatever you can do or dream you can begin it. Boldness has genius, power and magic in it" Goethe

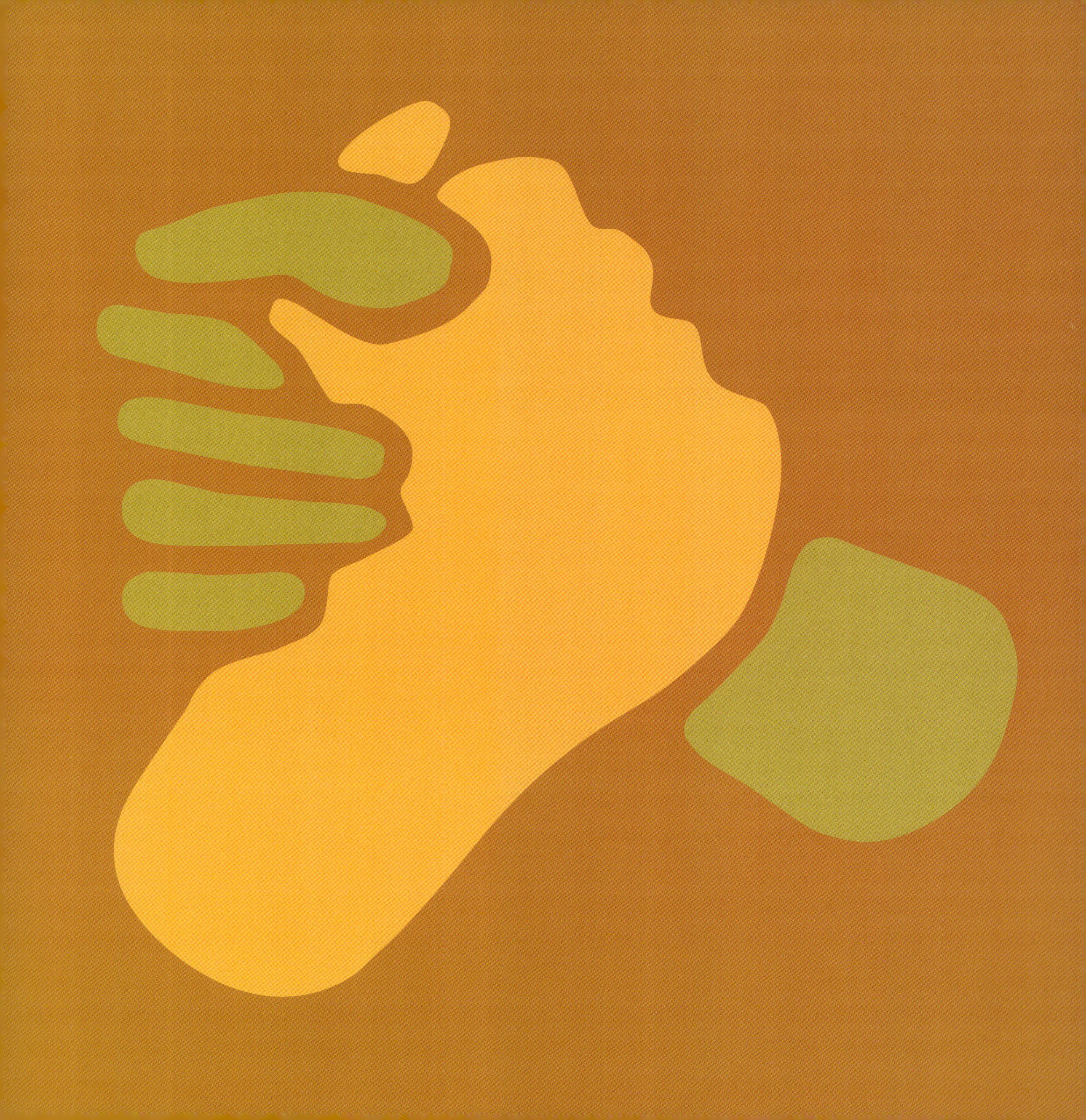

Tolerance 48

Developing tolerance through respect of others is a key skill for building your best self as well as compassion and understanding for the world in general.

The principle of separate realities is a mouthful, but an important principle to embrace if we are to fully build our best selves. Simply put, we all live independently, and our brains work separately from each other in their own worlds. By avoiding any dangerous assumption that other people may think the same as us we do, we can quickly learn respect for other people's lives. We can all grow by accepting each other's differences.

Think about what you are going to say and ask yourself 'Will my words cause harm or good for the person you are talking to?'

Once you have truly accepted other people's realities, that their lives are indeed their lives, and lived alongside others with different opinions and views, you will find humility. You will find a world where we have all been through, or are going to go through, the major traumas of life and death events. This **common bond** is unifying and builds great inner confidence with this knowledge.

"It's one of the greatest gifts you can give yourself: to forgive. Forgive everybody." Maya Angelou

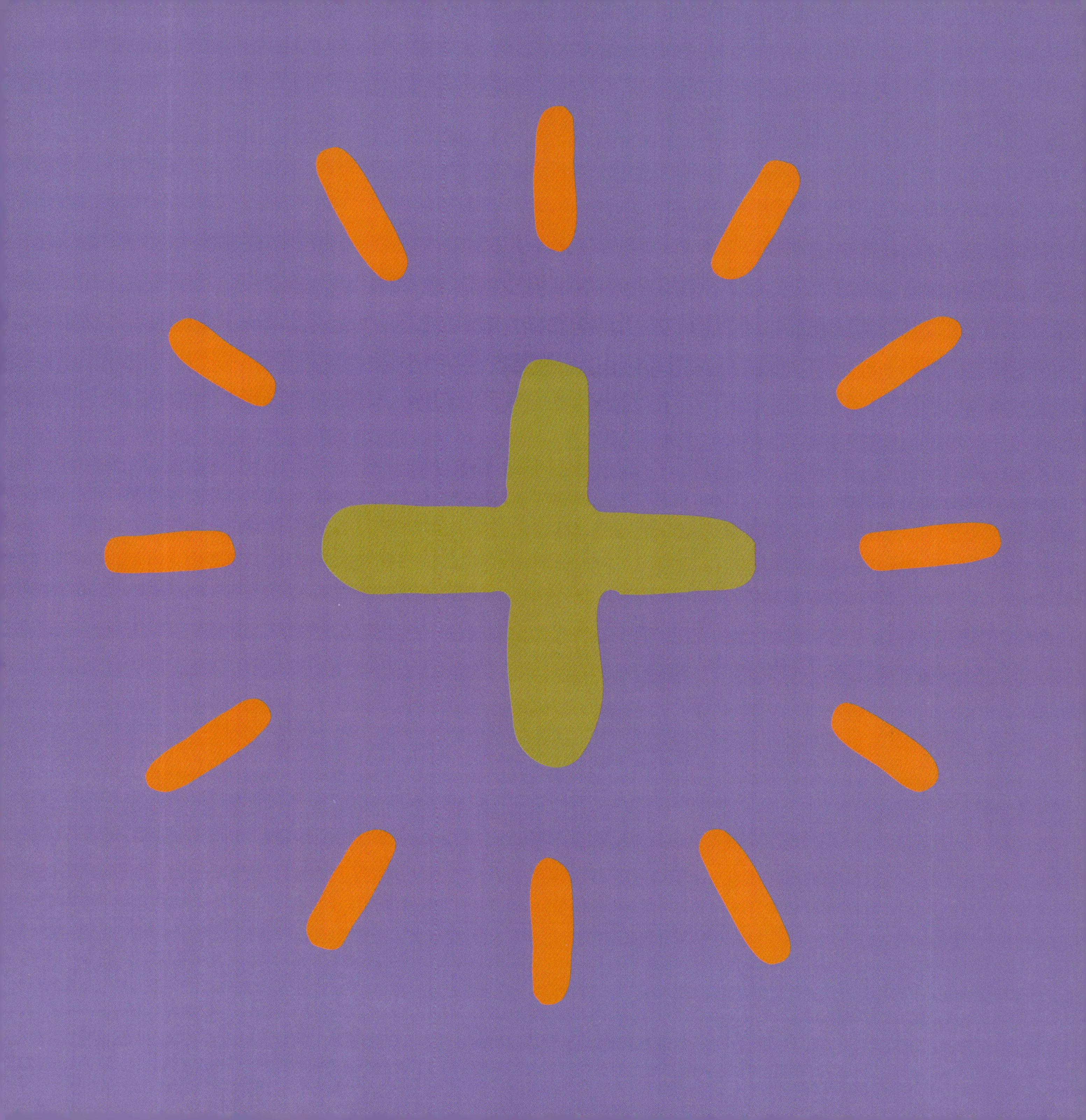

✚ Confidence 49

Key to a strong sense of self esteem is a greater sense of your social abilities and a greater emotional intelligence with the growth in personal confidence.

Finding a balanced sense of self esteem gives you the personal confidence to do more things in your life, with all the positive benefits these actions bring, such as broader social circles and more interesting social activity. It is **a positive spiral** that just keeps getting better.

Find a small task you dread doing and ask yourself, 'Why do I fear doing this?' When you have found sufficient answers and understand them, challenge them one at a time until you can carry out this task. You can build the challenges up each time you repeat the cycle.

Learning about yourself and learning your strengths as a human being will release a **personal freedom** to do stuff you might not otherwise do. The challenge and act of doing things out of your comfort zone, things you may have doubted yourself doing has so many benefits socially and internally. The twist is that until you get up and try these things you really don't know how they feel. I dare you.

"If my mind can conceive it, My heart can believe it, I know I can achieve it!" Jesse Jackson

“Everybody is different, thinks differently and acts differently. Until we learn to respect this and a respect for ourselves, it is far harder to move through life.”

“If I had to choose the most important word in the world right now it would be kindness”

7 Summary

Kindness costs nothing. It can be the smallest act, but it is also the glue that builds all of the best parts of all of us and all of civilisation.

The Tree of Self Esteem is about mindwork, turning thoughts into action, having the courage to get out of your comfort zone, acts of kindness, learning to give and take, finding equality and learning how other people might feel.

This is the big tree in the forest here. It is the stuff of peace, love and a wonderful world.

But for the purposes of this small and humble text, considerate behaviour, kind acts, greater understanding and tolerance are our start and finish to a better life and a rock solid wellbeing.

You never know, from small acorns...

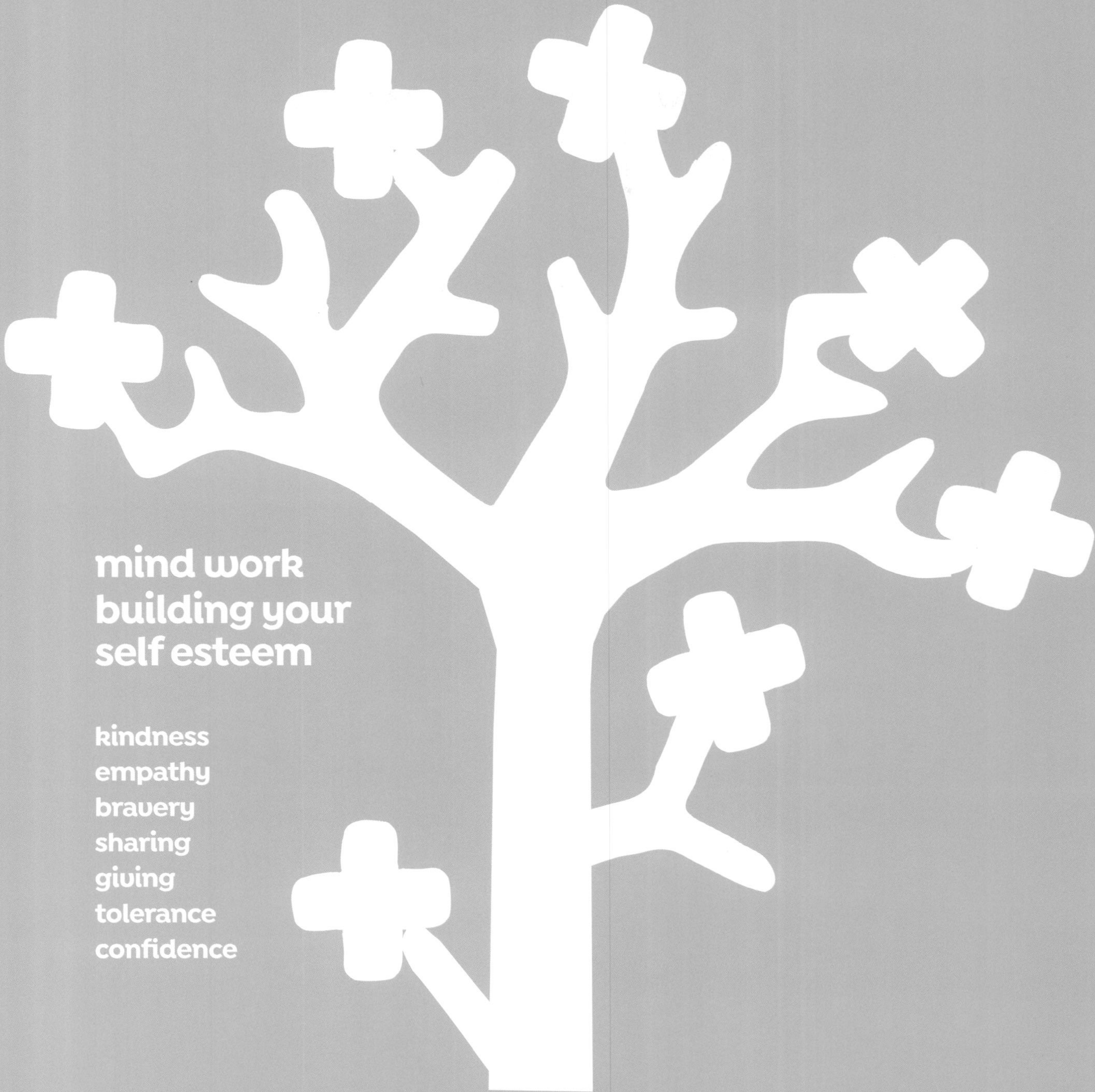

mind work building your self esteem

kindness
empathy
bravery
sharing
giving
tolerance
confidence

“Your mind is the most complicated thing in the universe. Learn to love it and amazing things happen”

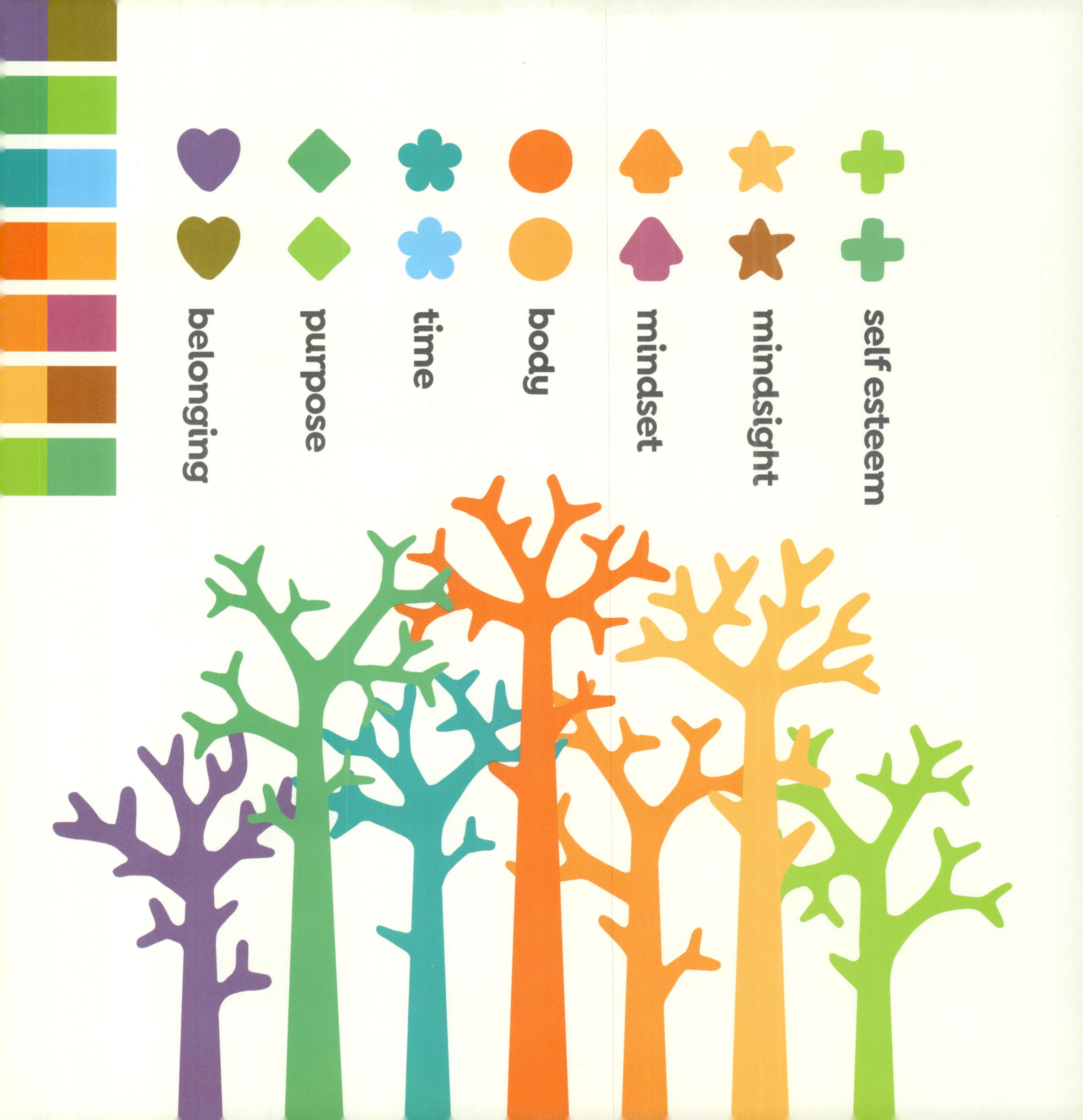
belonging
purpose
time
body
mindset
mindsight
self esteem

“Try using a notebook to keep a record of your thoughts, keep it honest, keep asking questions and keep going back to it. This record is great motivation”

Keeping a track – your notes

belonging

your personal challenge(s)
e.g. getting up and out and being more sociable.

purpose

your personal challenge(s)
e.g. puting some time aside for creative activity for yourself.

time

your personal challenge(s)
e.g. making sure you find more me time or some patience.

body

your personal challenge(s)
e.g. reduce alcohol or stop eating processed food for a week.

mindset

your personal challenge(s)
e.g. setting your mindset to 'can do' for a time.

mindsight

your personal challenge(s)
e.g. make a list of 3 good things about the day every evening.

self esteem

your personal challenge(s)
e.g. undertake a random act of kindness every day for a week.

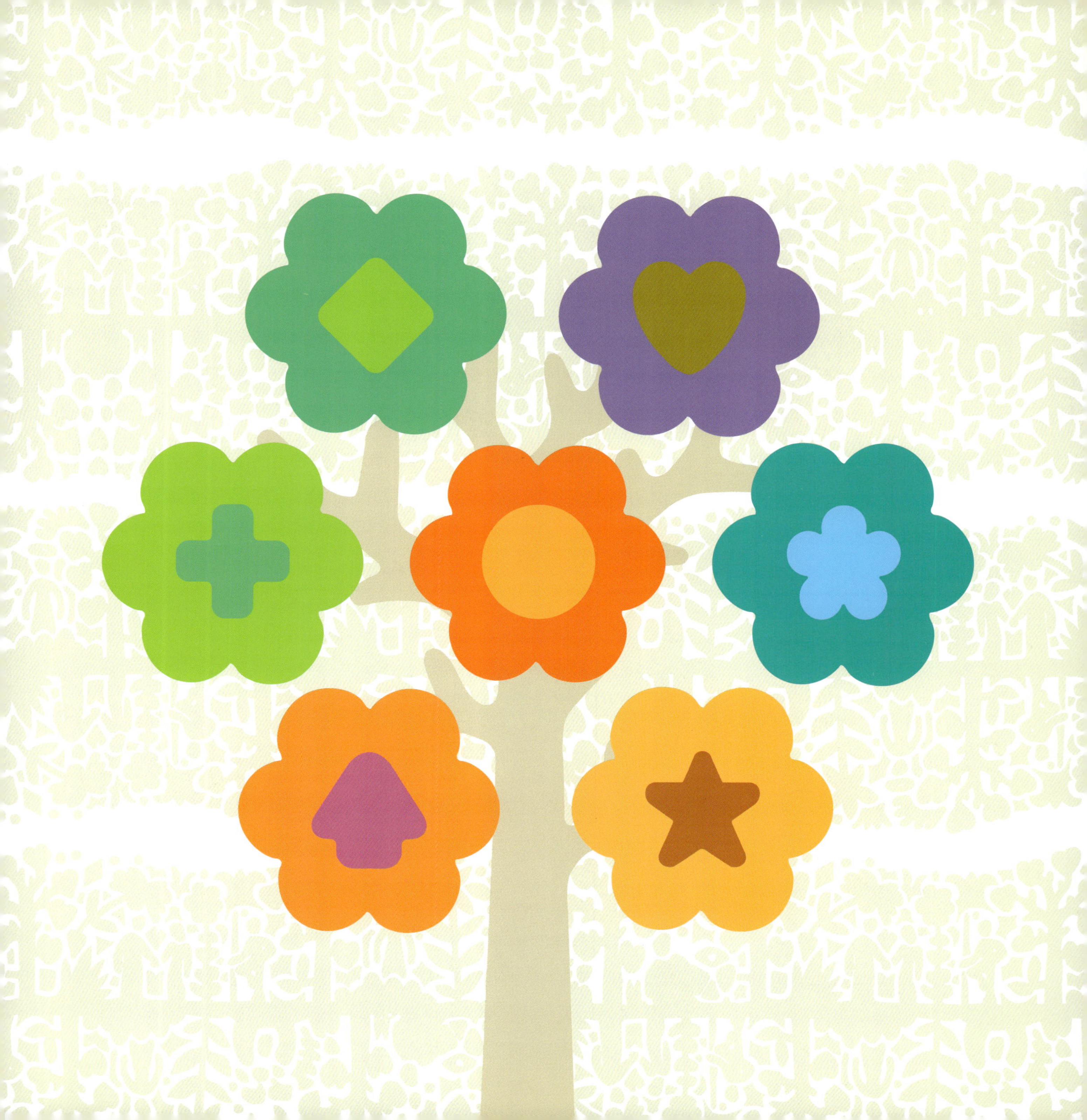

In other words

In order to create a simple system, the words of the magic forest were often chosen, from a short list of words, to mean the same or something similar.

01 Love
Care
02 Friends
Friendship
03 Family
04 Honesty
05 Talk
Communication
06 Tribe
Community
07 Belonging
08 Playing
09 Living
Life
Doing
Lifestyle
10 Wisdom
11 Own
Responsibility
Trust
12 Challenge
Goal
13 Commit
14 Purpose
15 Be
Being
16 Quiet
Peace
17 Centre
18 Joy
Rewards
Recreation
Giggle
Laugh
Sing
19 Sleep
Rest
20 Patience
21 Now
22 Needs
23 Move
Exercise
Movement
24 Drive
Motivation
25 Eat
Nutrition
26 Energy
Vitality
27 Drink
Hydration
28 Balance
29 Attitude
30 Positivity
31 Humility
Thank
32 Think
Thinking
Considered
Thoughts
33 Control
34 Pattern
35 Safety
Home
36 Belief
Values
Believe
Opinions
37 Magic
Reward
38 Inheritance
39 Happiness
40 Hope
41 Love of Self
Self Love
42 Perception
See
Watch
Observe
43 Kindness
44 Empathy
45 Sharing
Inspire
Teach
46 Giving
Hug
47 Bravery
Courage
48 Tolerance
Acceptance
49 Confidence
Esteem

About the author

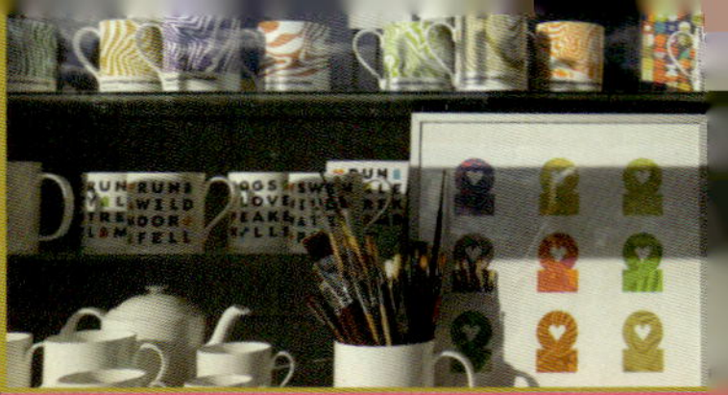

Si Homfray is an artist, designer, professional creative, adventurer and author based in the Peak District.

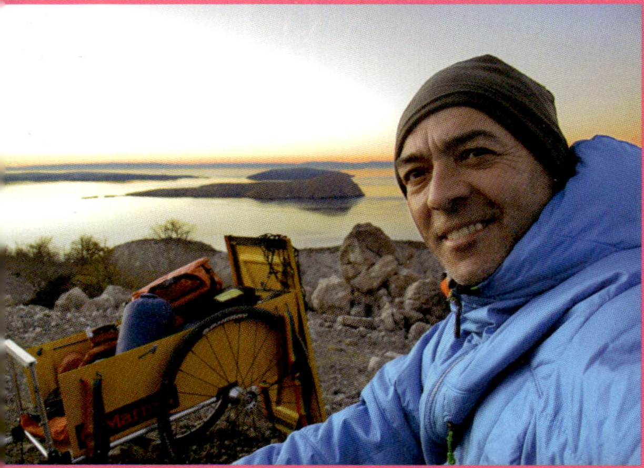

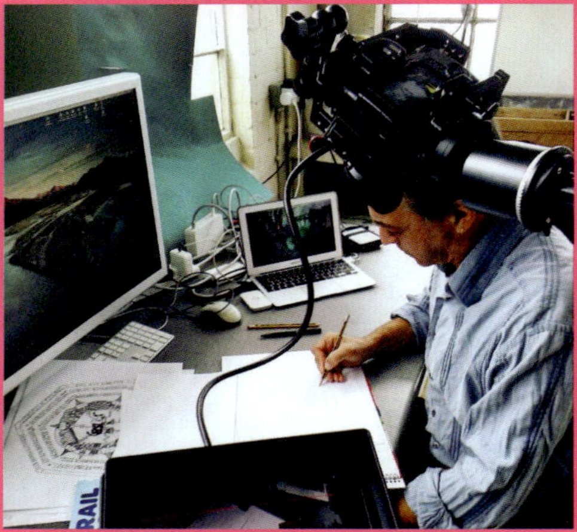

Si owns and runs Park Designs, which was set up, after a lifetime living in the Peak District, as an outlet for Si's artistic expressions of the National Park.

After a career working in graphic design with many of the UKs loved businesses, organisations and brands who share a care for the natural world, he is now finding and producing his own style of art and quality gifts featuring wellbeing, the National Parks and his favourite open spaces around the UK.

His many travels and varied physical activities in the Park combined with a curiosity to find new ways of interpreting information are leading to some exciting new themes around wellbeing and the natural world.

He is currently focussed on how this immersion can help generate personal growth, inner calm and a strong foundation for a more solid wellbeing and richer life.

we all need a big passion, a reason to be.
we all need a big friend, to share the troubles of the day.
we all need a big giggle, the reward that loosens our shoulders.
we all need a little care, the nutrients that fertilise our soil.
we all need a little smile, the turned corners of a strangers gift.
we all need a little love, the shared feelings that bond our very being.
we all need to hug, to closen ties to our humanity.
we all need a place, to disappear and return refreshed.
we all need to know warmth, the wrap of a home.
but above all… we all need to consider the other.
we all need to be together.
we all need to keep being kind, thoughtful consideration and generosity of spirit.
and… we all need to keep being We.

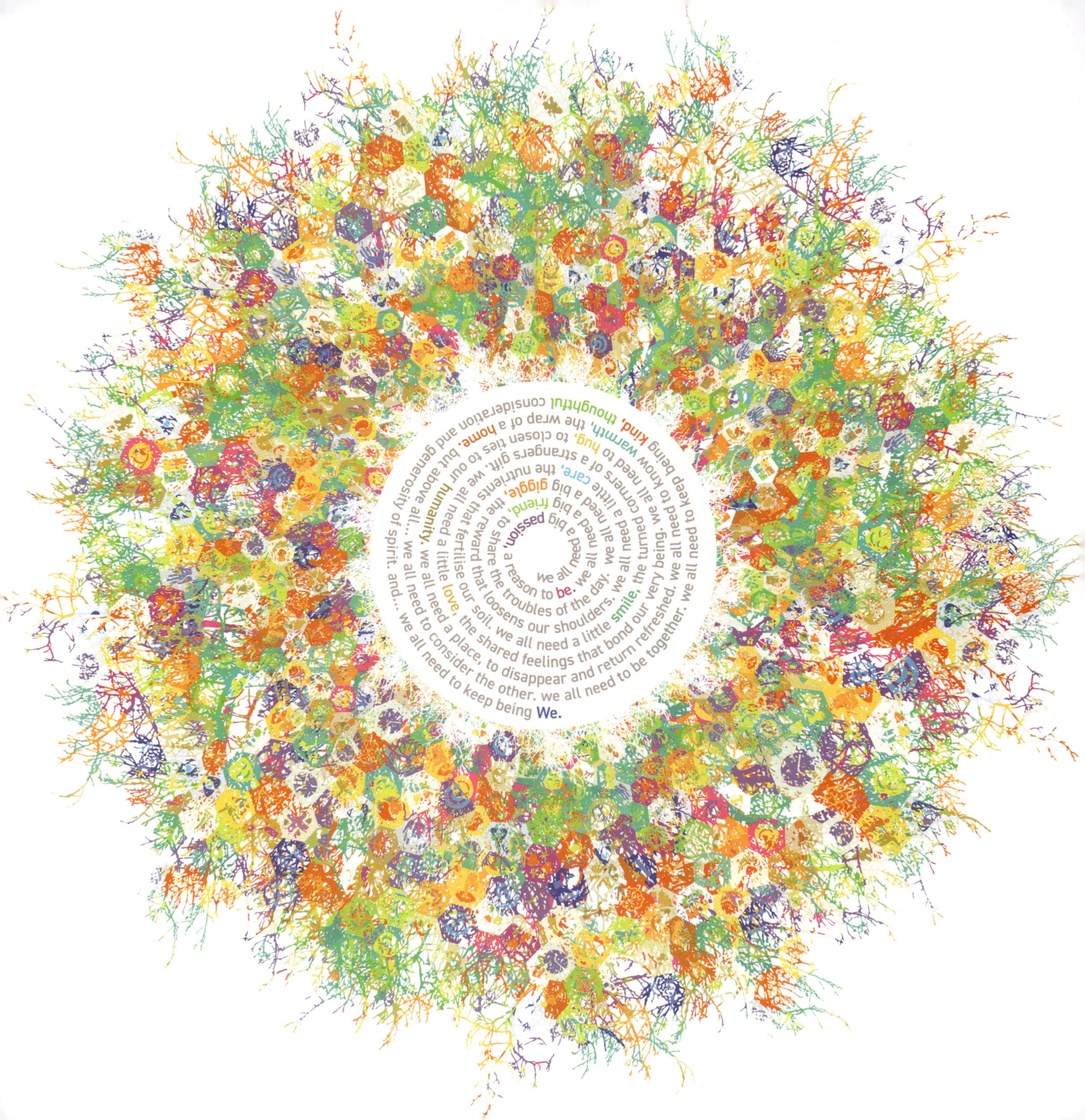
we all need a big passion, a reason to be. we all need a big friend, to share the troubles of the day. we all need a big giggle, the reward that loosens our shoulders. we all need a little care, the nutrients that fertilise our soil. we all need a little smile, the turned corners of a strangers gift. we all need a little love, the shared feelings that bond our very being. we all need to hug, to closen ties to our humanity. we all need a place, to disappear and return refreshed. we all need to know warmth, the wrap of a home. but above all... we all need to consider the other. we all need to be together. we all need to keep being kind, thoughtful consideration and generosity of spirit. and... we all need to keep being We.

Bibilography

A short list of some of the books and media that I have read over the years that have influenced my thinking, the opinions and some of the detail in this book.

The Art of Happiness (Riverhead, 1998, ISBN 1-57322-111-2)

Marcus Buckingham Now, Discover Your Strengths (with Donald O. Clifton; The Free Press, 2001)

Laing, R.D. (1960) The Divided Self: An Existential Study in Sanity and Madness.

Laing, R.D. (1967) The Politics of Experience and the Bird of Paradise. Harmondsworth: Penguin.

Gilbert, Paul (2010). The Compassionate Mind: A New Approach to Life's Challenges. Oakland, CA: New Harbinger Publications. ISBN 9781572248403

1995: Emotional Intelligence: Why It Can Matter More Than IQ, Bantam Books. ISBN 978-0-553-38371-3

Kahneman, Daniel (2011). Thinking, Fast and Slow. Farrar, Straus and Giroux. ISBN 978-0374275631

Carl Jung - Memories, Dreams, Reflections 0-00-654027-9 (Fontana Press edition)

You Can Be Happy No Matter What: Five Principles Your Therapist Never Told You. New World Library, 1997. ISBN 1-57731-064-0.

I'm OK – You're OK - Thomas Anthony Harris. - 978-0060724276

Anthony Storr - The Integrity of the Personality (1961) ISBN 978-0-345-37585-8

Herman Hesse - Steppenwolf (originally Der Steppenwolf) 0-312-27867-5

www.scientificamerican.com - https://www.scientificamerican.com/article/100-trillion-connections/

Patch Adams (1998) - The true story of a heroic man, Hunter "Patch" Adams, determined to become a medical doctor because he enjoys helping people - Starring Robin Williams

Haston, Dougal (1974). The Eiger. London: Cassell. ISBN 0-304-29373-3.

Jurek, Scott; Friedman, Steve (2012). Eat & Run: My Unlikely Journey to Ultramarathon Greatness. Houghton Mifflin Harcourt. ISBN 978-0547569659.

McDougall, Christopher (2009). Born to Run: A Hidden Tribe, Superathletes, and the Greatest Race the World Has Never Seen. New York: Knopf. ISBN 978-0-307-26630-9.

Hofmann SG (2011). "An Introduction to Modern CBT". Psychological Solutions to Mental Health Problems. Chichester, UK: Wiley-Blackwell. ISBN 978-0470971758.

I Know Why the Caged Bird Sings - 1969 - Maya Angelou - 978-0860685111

“You could use the selector wheel to go round every aspect of your wellbeing... again and again”

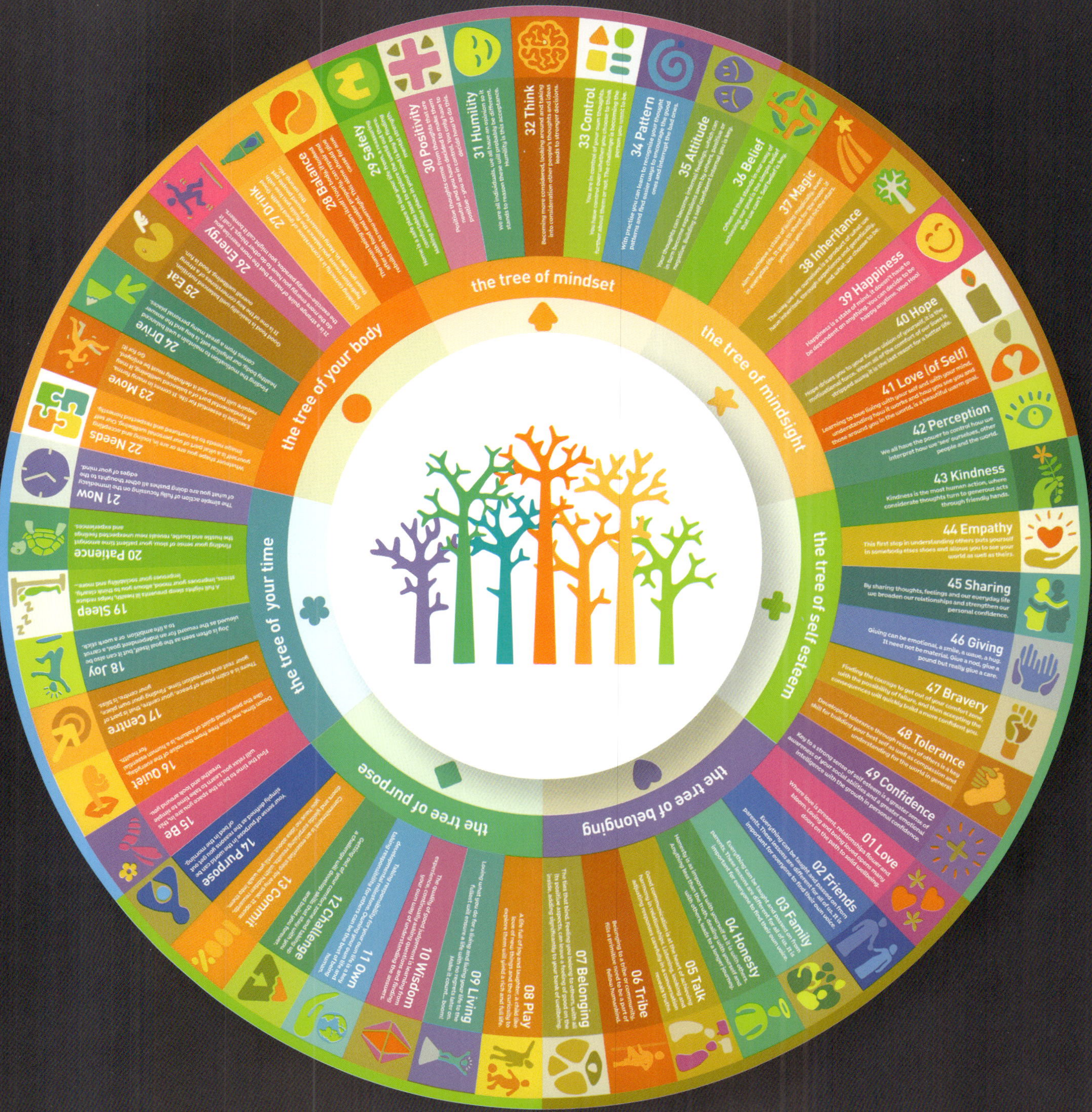

the tree of mindset
the tree of mindsight
the tree of self esteem
the tree of belonging
the tree of purpose
the tree of your time
the tree of your body
01 Love
02 Friends
03 Family
04 Honesty
05 Talk
06 Tribe
07 Belonging
08 Play
09 Living
10 Wisdom
11 Own
12 Challenge
13 Commit
14 Purpose
15 Be
16 Quiet
17 Centre
18 Joy
19 Sleep
20 Patience
21 Now
22 Needs
23 Move
24 Drive
25 Eat
26 Energy
27 Drink
28 Balance
29 Safety
30 Positivity
31 Humility
32 Think
33 Control
34 Pattern
35 Attitude
36 Belief
37 Magic
38 Inheritance
39 Happiness
40 Hope
41 Love (of Self)
42 Perception
43 Kindness
44 Empathy
45 Sharing
46 Giving
47 Bravery
48 Tolerance
49 Confidence

Magic Beans

It's a kind'a magic!

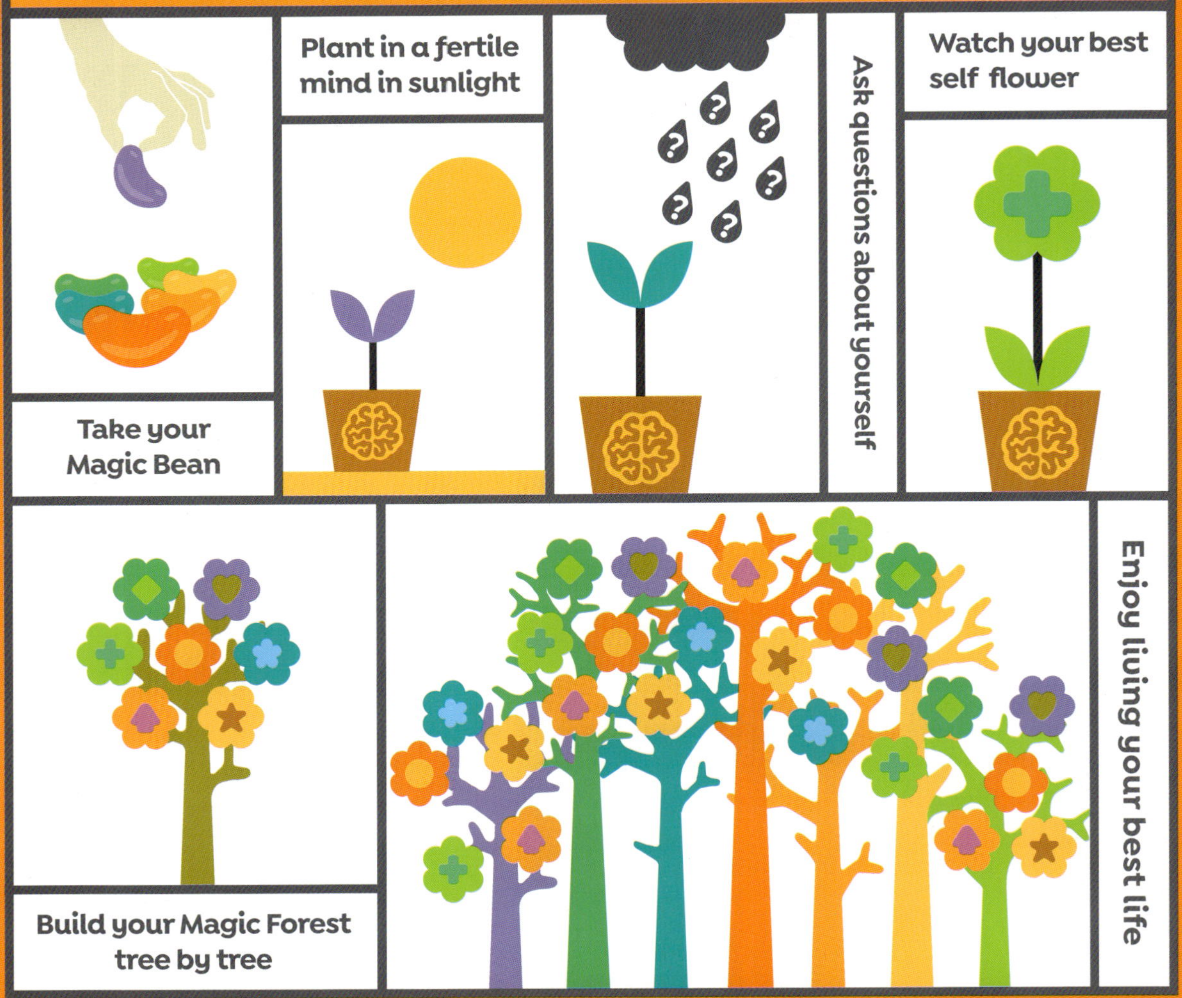

Take your Magic Bean
Plant in a fertile mind in sunlight
Ask questions about yourself
Watch your best self flower
Build your Magic Forest tree by tree
Enjoy living your best life

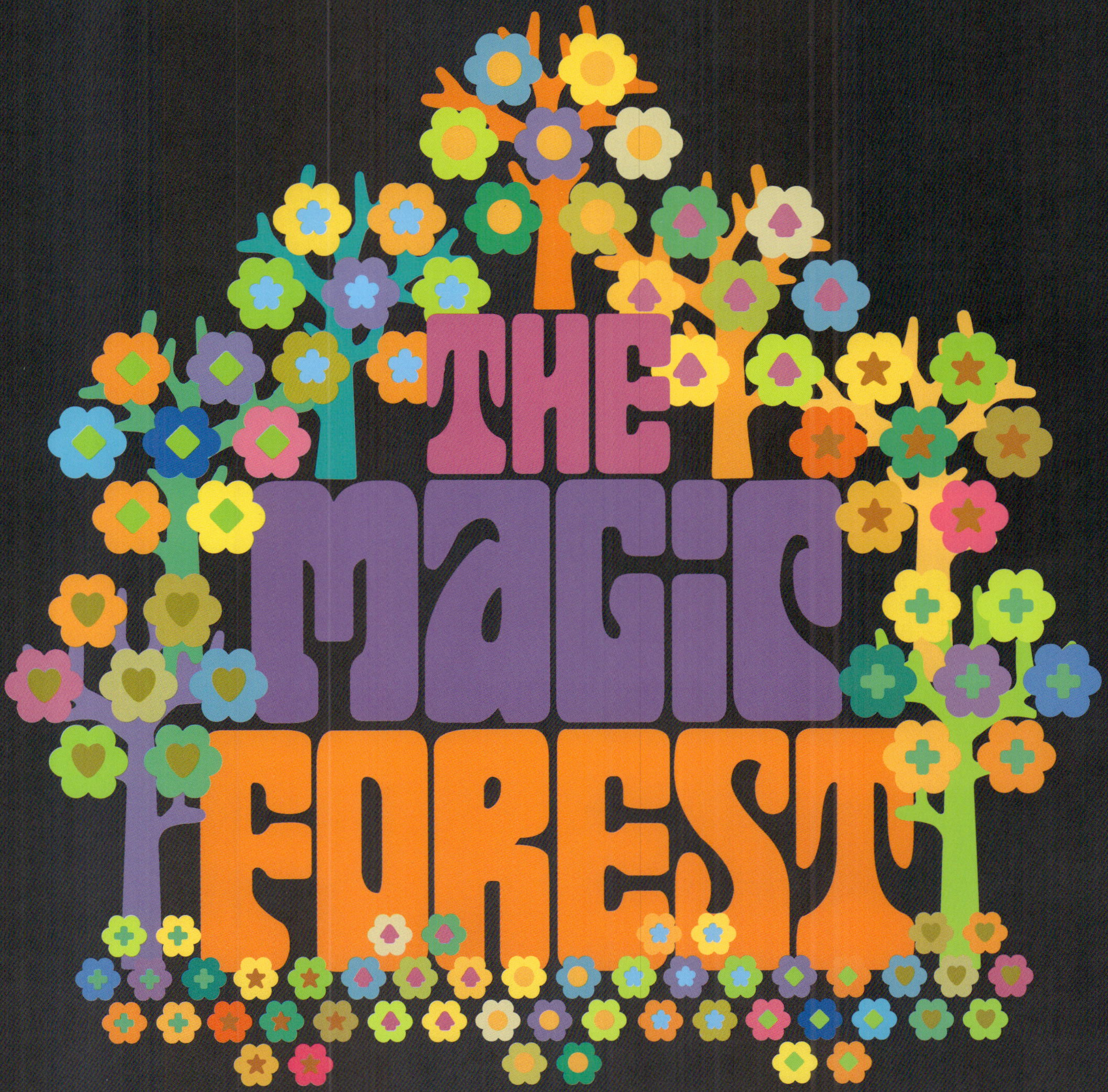
THE
MAGIC
FOREST

7 trees

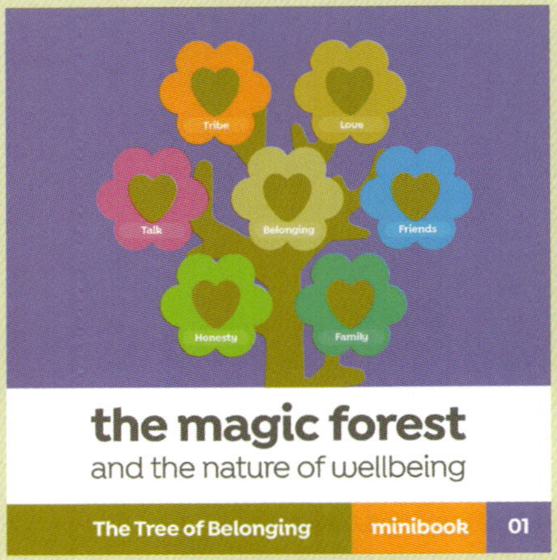

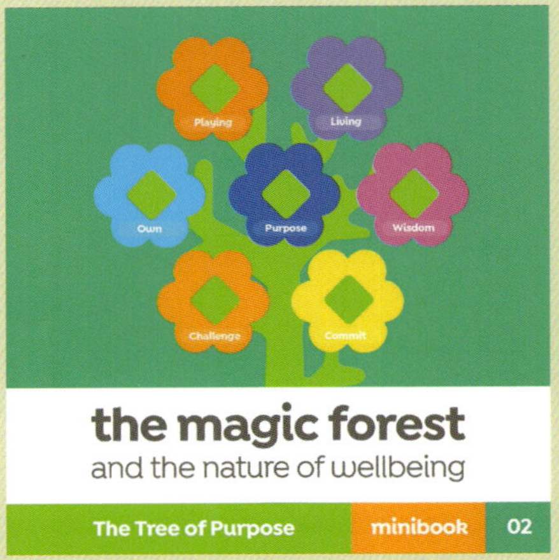

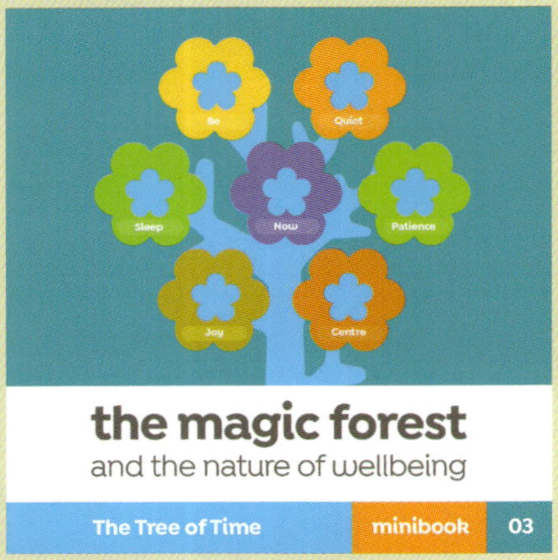

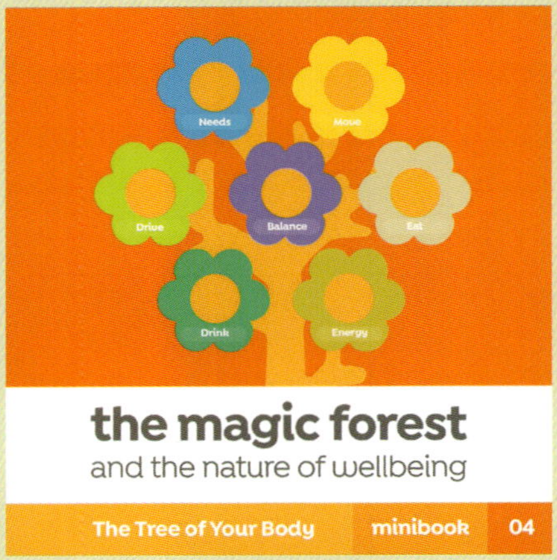

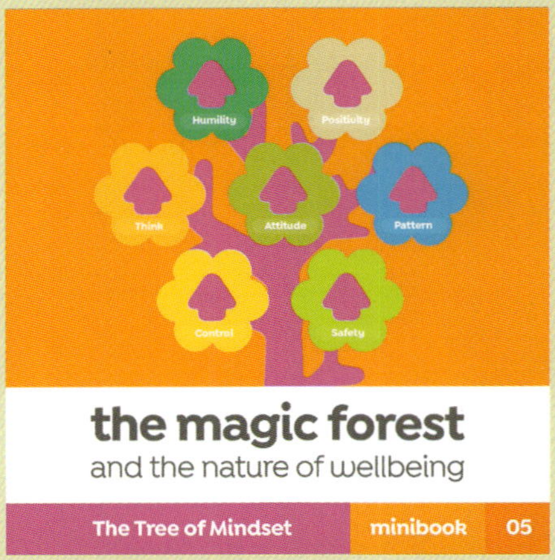

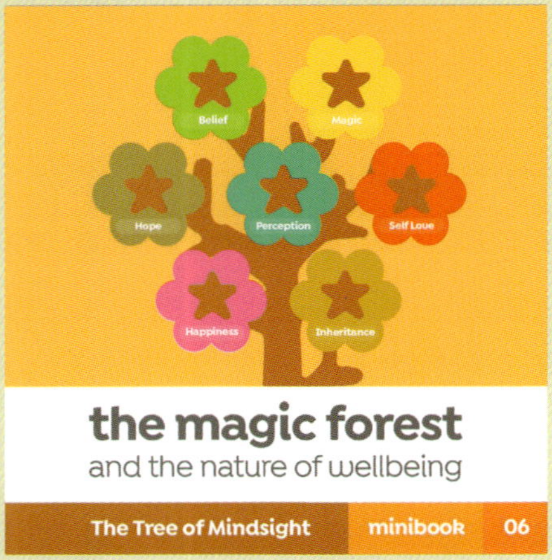

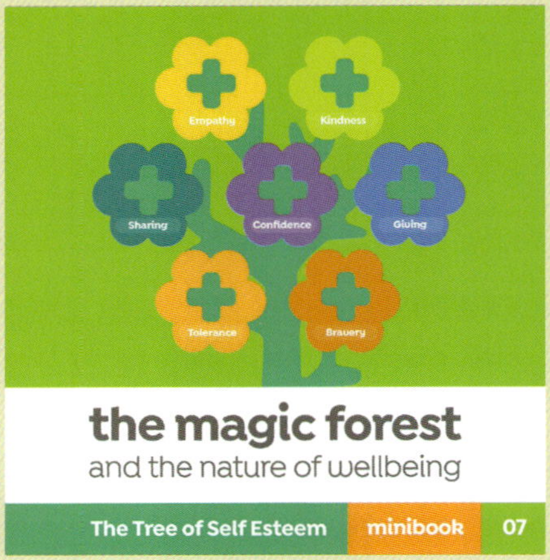

7 mini books

“The wonderful thing about this system is that you are in total control of what you do, how you do it and when.”

“A key challenge for this wellbeing system is to find the right answers for you. Once you have found a few of your answers you start to feel great and keep building”

Overview

The Tree of Belonging

Building your sense of belonging through:

01 Love
02 Friends
03 Family
04 Honesty
05 Talk
06 Tribe
07 Belonging

The Tree of Purpose

Building your sense of purpose through:

08 Playing
09 Living
10 Wisdom
11 Own
12 Challenge
13 Commit
14 Purpose

The Tree of Time

Rest, recreation and building your sense of time through:

15 Be
16 Quiet
17 Centre
18 Joy
19 Sleep
20 Patience
21 Now

The Tree of Your Body

Building your physical you through:

22 Needs
23 Move
24 Drive
25 Eat
26 Energy
27 Drink
28 Balance

The Tree of Mindsetting

Learning control for your mind through:

29 Safety
30 Positivity
31 Humility
32 Think
33 Control
34 Pattern
35 Attitude

The Tree of Mindsight

Building how you see your world and others' through:

36 Belief
37 Magic
38 Inheritance
39 Happiness
40 Hope
41 Self Love
42 Perception

The Tree of Self Esteem

Building your self esteem through:

43 Kindness
44 Empathy
45 Sharing
46 Giving
47 Bravery
48 Tolerance
49 Confidence

The Magic Forest & the nature of wellbeing

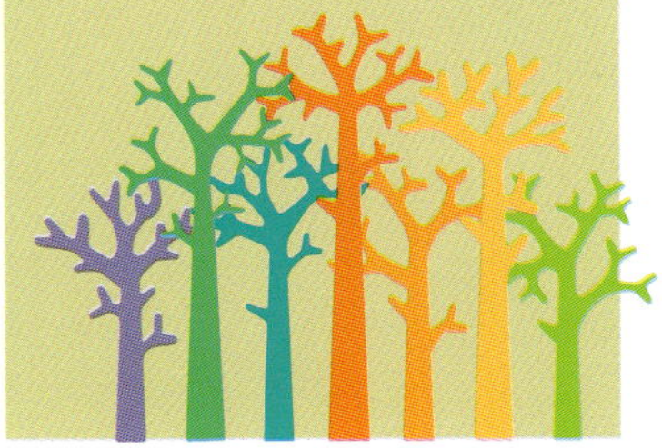